Small Animal Fluid Therapy

Small Animal Fluid Therapy

Edward Cooper (coordinating author)

The Ohio State University, USA

Julien Guillaumin

Colorado State University, USA

Jiwoong Her

The Ohio State University, USA

Page Yaxley

The Ohio State University, USA

and

Anda Young

The Ohio State University, USA

CABI

CABI is a trading name of CAB International

CABI
Nosworthy Way
Wallingford
Oxfordshire OX10 8DE
UK

Tel: +44 (0)1491 832111
E-mail: info@cabi.org
Website: www.cabi.org

CABI
200 Portland Street
Boston
MA 02114
USA

Tel: +1 (617)682-9015
E-mail: cabi-nao@cabi.org

A catalogue record for this book is available from the British Library, London, UK.

Library of Congress Cataloging-in-Publication Data

Names: Cooper, Edward S., 1976- author.
Title: Small animal fluid therapy / Edward Cooper, VMD, MS, DACVECC, The Ohio State University, Columbus, OH, USA, Julien Guillaumin, DVM, DACVECC, DECVECC, Colorado State University, Fort Collins, CO, USA, Jiwoong Her, DVM, MS, DACVECC, The Ohio State University, Columbus, OH, USA, Page Yaxley, DVM, DACVECC, The Ohio State University, Columbus, OH, USA, Anda Young, DVM, MS, DACVECC, The Ohio State University, Columbus, OH, USA.
Description: Oxfordshire, UK ; Boston, MA, USA : CAB International, [2022] | Includes bibliographical references and index. | Summary: "Fluid therapy is one of the most important aspects of therapy in veterinary medicine. In this book the authors provide guidelines for the safe implementation of fluid therapy in clinical practice"-- Provided by publisher.
Identifiers: LCCN 2022032405 (print) | LCCN 2022032406 (ebook) | ISBN 9781789243383 (hardback) | ISBN 9781789243390 (ePDF) | ISBN 9781789243406 (ePub)
Subjects: LCSH: Pet medicine. | Veterinary fluid therapy. | Dogs--Diseases--Treatment. | Cats--Diseases--Treatment.
Classification: LCC SF981 .C66 2022 (print) | LCC SF981 (ebook) | DDC 636.089--dc23/eng/20220822
LC record available at https://lccn.loc.gov/2022032405
LC ebook record available at https://lccn.loc.gov/2022032406

ISBN-13: 9781789243383 (hardback)
9781789243390 (ePDF)
9781789243406 (ePub)

DOI: 10.1079/9781789243406.0000

Commissioning Editor: Alexandra Lainsbury
Editorial Assistant: Emma McCann
Production Editor: Shankari Wilford

Typeset by SPi, Pondicherry, India
Printed and bound in the UK by Severn, Gloucester

Contents

About the authors vii

Foreword ix
Edward Cooper – Coordinating author

1 Introduction: Importance and Role of Fluid Therapy in Small Animal Practice 1
Edward Cooper

2 Body Fluid Compartments 3
Edward Cooper

3 Fluid Types – Crystalloids 10
Edward Cooper

4i–ii Fluid Types: Colloids

4i Synthetic Colloids 18
Anda Young

4ii Natural Colloids 26
Julien Guillaumin

5 Routes of Fluid Administration 33
Edward Cooper

6i–iii General Approach to Fluid Therapy (Application and Monitoring)

6i Resuscitation Fluid Therapy 41
Edward Cooper

6ii Replacement Fluid Therapy 54
Julien Guillaumin

6iii Maintenance Fluid Therapy 63
Jiwoong Her

7i–iv Fluid Supplementation

7i Dextrose Supplementation 68
Edward Cooper

7ii Potassium Supplementation 73
Page Yaxley

7iii Calcium and Phosphorus Supplementation 81
Anda Young

7iv Magnesium Supplementation 91
Julien Guillaumin

8i–ix Selected Clinical Circumstances and Case Scenarios

8i Special Considerations for Patients Experiencing Hemorrhage/Trauma 95
Edward Cooper

8ii Special Considerations for Septic Patients 103
Julien Guillaumin

8iii Impact of Heart Disease on Fluid Therapy 107
Jiwoong Her

8iv Impact of Renal Disease on Fluid Therapy 110
Anda Young

8v Anesthesia/Perioperative Fluid Considerations 115
Jiwoong Her

8vi Management of Hypernatremia and Hyponatremia 119
Julien Guillaumin

8vii Approach to Fluid Therapy in Patients with Hypoproteinemia 123
Julien Guillaumin

8viii Special Considerations in Neonates/Pediatrics 126
Page Yaxley

8ix Special Considerations in Cats 133
Anda Young

Index 141

About the Authors

Edward Cooper, VMD, MS, DACVECC (coordinating author)
Professor – Clinical
Small Animal Emergency and Critical Care – Head of Service
The Ohio State University College of Veterinary Medicine, 601 Vernon Tharp Street, Columbus, OH, 43085, USA
Email: cooper.1697@osu.edu

Julien Guillaumin, DVM, DACVECC, DECVECC
Associate Professor – Critical Care Unit
Colorado State University College of Veterinary Medicine and Biomedical Sciences, 1350 Centre Ave, Fort Collins, CO 80521, USA
Email: julien.guillaumin@colostate.edu

Jiwoong Her, DVM, MS, DACVECC
Assistant Professor – Clinical
Small Animal Emergency and Critical Care
The Ohio State University College of Veterinary Medicine, 601 Vernon Tharp Street, Columbus, OH, 43085, USA
Email: her.22@osu.edu

Page Yaxley, DVM, DACVECC
Associate Professor – Clinical
Small Animal Emergency and Critical Care
The Ohio State University College of Veterinary Medicine, 601 Vernon Tharp Street, Columbus, OH, 43085, USA
Email: yaxley.1@osu.edu

Anda Young, DVM, MS, DACVECC
Assistant Professor – Clinical
Small Animal Emergency and Critical Care
The Ohio State University College of Veterinary Medicine, 601 Vernon Tharp Street, Columbus, OH, 43085, USA
Email: young.2633@osu.edu

Foreword

Fluid therapy constitutes an important aspect of patient care in a variety of small animal practices. However, decisions related to the type, volume, and rate of fluid administration remain a daunting undertaking for many in veterinary medicine, especially veterinary students and new practitioners. Ideally there would be a single fluid therapy plan that would suit each and every patient, but unfortunately this does not exist. Compounded by the potential for fluids to have limitations and adverse effects, it becomes even more important to tailor a plan to meet the patient's needs.

In an effort to help demystify some of these concepts, and reach beyond the students we teach each year, we sought to create a resource that would provide a practical framework of background and application. We sought to highlight the building blocks without getting too lost in the theory, pathophysiology, or minutiae that can be more distracting than insightful. Finally, we sought to help the reader achieve the ultimate goal of developing a fluid therapy plan – optimize the benefits and minimize the risks for each individual patient. It is a delicate balance to strike. And while there are many ways to approach fluid therapy, we hope the information, case examples, and practice calculations provided here prove useful in that endeavor.

Edward Cooper, VMD, MS, DACVECC
Coordinating Author

1 Introduction: Importance and Role of Fluid Therapy in Small Animal Practice

EDWARD COOPER

The Ohio State University, Columbus, Ohio, USA

Veterinary medicine has become progressively broader in its scope, while simultaneously much more advanced and specialized in its application. From the primary care veterinary clinic to secondary and tertiary care facilities, fluid therapy constitutes a major component of patient management and therapeutic intervention. A variety of clinical circumstances could warrant fluid administration, including replacing dehydration, providing fluids during anesthesia, resuscitation of the patient in shock, daily fluid needs, etc. The patient may be healthy or ill, young or old; it could have heart disease, kidney disease, obesity, or any number of underlying disease processes. As such, decisions related to fluid therapy can prove daunting to many practitioners when faced with the task of answering the cardinal questions of fluid administration:

- What type of fluids should I use?
- What is the best route of delivery?
- How much should I give?
- How quickly (or slowly) should I deliver those fluids?

In an ideal world, there would be one type of fluid administered the same way at a rate based on one magical formula that is perfect for every patient. Unfortunately, that magical formula does not exist, and each fluid type and route of delivery has potential benefits and drawbacks specific to the patient and the clinical situation. Some patients need to be given fluids more quickly in order to be effective, while others should receive them more slowly to decrease risk of harm. Numerous factors need to be considered, and so there cannot (and should not) be a "one-size-fits-all" approach when formulating a fluid therapy plan. It should be tailored to the patient at hand to optimize the impact and minimize any adverse effects that fluids may have.

What follows in this text is the background information, as well as the practical application, to help practitioners achieve this goal. The sections and material have been designed to provide the framework to make fluid decisions for any individual patient, and not just provide a cookbook for all patients. In Chapter 2, body fluid compartments will be presented. While not the most glamorous, it is important to appreciate how water, electrolytes, and colloids are normally distributed across the body, so that it then becomes clearer what happens to fluids after they are given. These relationships are important to better understand what type of fluid to choose as well, which sets the stage for Chapters 3 and 4. Fluids are more than just water, with varying electrolyte compositions, effects on acid–base balance, and distributive properties in the body. Achieving an understanding of the different fluid types (crystalloid and colloids) allows for better understanding of their implications and potential applications, as well as adverse effects and contraindications.

Deciding the route of administration is another important component of developing a fluid therapy plan. Chapter 5 provides an overview of these considerations from use of a central or peripheral venous catheter, to intraosseous catheter placement, to administration of subcutaneous fluids, to fluids delivered enterally. Each of these routes has potential benefits and drawbacks which will be impacted by factors related to the patient's clinical condition, the reason fluid is needed, and whether hospitalized care is possible.

DOI: 10.1079/9781789243406.0001

Not until the type of fluid and route of administration have been selected can the total dose and rate of delivery be determined. Decisions regarding volume and rate should be made based on several factors, and so Chapter 6 provides the framework for establishing a general approach based on patient needs. Is the patient in need of resuscitation (rapid expansion of the vascular volume), replacement (restoring interstitial volume from dehydration and ongoing losses), and/or administration of maintenance fluid (providing basic daily water and electrolytes)? Depending on which of these is the target, starting fluids rates can then be calculated. Ongoing clinical assessment and monitoring of how the patient responds is essential in order to make necessary adjustments to the fluid therapy plan and ensure that the goals are being met.

Beyond provision of the fluids themselves, many patients need additional supplementation of electrolytes or supportive additives like dextrose. Fluid therapy can provide the conduit for delivering these supplements, though it can also contribute to their derangements. To that end, discussion of how electrolyte abnormalities may impact the patient, when fluid additives might be needed, and how to perform calculations for appropriate and safe administration, is covered in Chapter 7.

While a general approach will work for most patients, there are many circumstances that could impact fluid therapy choices independently of the absolute fluid needs. It would not be possible to account for every caveat; however, Chapter 8 endeavors to address many of the more common situations that may prompt adjustment to fluid administration. Whether the patient has experienced trauma or sepsis, has kidney or heart disease, has changes in free water or loss of protein, needs to undergo anesthesia, is newborn or pediatric, or is a cat rather than a dog, can significantly impact all aspects of fluid administration.

Bringing together all these pieces is important to unravel some of the mystery and complexities of fluid administration. To help achieve this, the concepts in this book are provided along with numerous calculations and case examples to make them as clinically applicable and user-friendly as possible. Through the combination of these things, hopefully it will become clear that, while there is no magical formula, fluid therapy essentially boils down to the following:

- Pick a fluid and route appropriate for the clinical situation.
- Give enough to meet the patient's needs, but try not to give too much.
- Give it as fast as you need to, but as slow as you can.

This text aims to provide the building blocks needed to optimize the safety and efficacy of fluid therapy in a way that could be applied to any patient in order to achieve these goals.

2 Body Fluid Compartments

EDWARD COOPER

The Ohio State University, Columbus, Ohio, USA

The first step toward building a fluid therapy plan involves thinking about how water, electrolytes, and colloids are distributed across the body, and the factors that govern their movement from one compartment to another. While the immediate clinical application of this may seem abstract, appreciating these relationships allows better understanding of what happens to fluids after they are administered. Knowing where they go, relative to where they are needed, will impact the type of fluid that may be selected, as well as how much may need to be given.

2.1 Total Body Water

Total body water reflects the percentage of body weight that is water versus "dry matter". In general, this has been determined to be approximately 60% in both adult dogs and cats (Stanton *et al.*, 1992; Wamberg *et al.*, 2002). However, there are several factors that may impact this overall distribution, including age, gender, and body condition. For example, neonates have closer to 80% total body water (MacIntire, 2008), whereas obese patients are more likely to have a lower percentage of body water compared with patients with normal body condition.

2.2 Body Fluid Compartments

Fluid within the body is divided into various compartments that are separated by different barriers which dictate the movement of water and solutes between them (Fig. 2.1 and Table 2.1). The largest of these is the **intracellular space**, comprising the fluid contained within cells. This constitutes approximately two-thirds of total body water, or 40% of body weight. Body fluids not contained within cells are considered to be part of the **extracellular space**, which is the remaining one-third of total body water, or 20% of body weight. The **cell membrane** is the principal barrier between these two compartments. The extracellular space is further divided into the **interstitial** and **intravascular** (plasma) compartments. The relative proportion of extracellular fluid in these compartments is estimated to be approximately three-quarters interstitial (or about 15% of body weight) and one-quarter intravascular (or 4–6% of body weight in dogs and 3–5% of body weight in cats) (Kohn and DiBartola, 2000). The endothelium, and more specifically the **endothelial surface layer** (ESL), is the principal barrier between these two compartments. It is important to note that while there are also red blood cells in the intravascular space, the water within them is technically considered part of the intracellular compartment. That is why the total blood volume (plasma plus red blood cells) is greater than what has been described for plasma alone. Reported total blood volumes for dogs is 8–9% of body weight, whereas cats have a smaller circulating volume relative to size with only 5–7% of body weight (Jain, 1986).

2.3 Movement between Intracellular and Extracellular Compartments

As previously indicated, the principal barrier between the intracellular and extracellular compartments is the cell membrane. This lipid bilayer is freely permeable to water but restricted to the movement of electrolytes and larger molecules like proteins unless they are actively transported. Further, these transport mechanisms (particularly the Na/K ATPase) function to maintain very different electrolyte compositions between these two compartments (Table 2.2). As a result, sodium is the predominant extracellular ion, whereas potassium is the predominant intracellular ion. These differences are essential to maintaining intracellular function, as well as extracellular homeostasis. However, the overall **osmolality** (reflecting the

DOI: 10.1079/9781789243406.0002

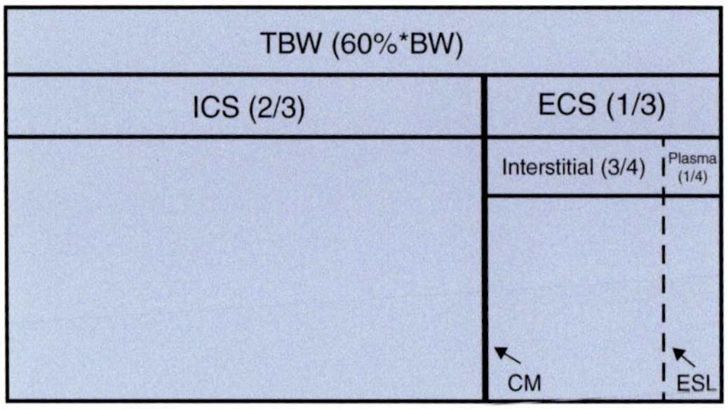

TBW: Total body water; BW: Body weight in kilograms; ICS: Intracellular fluid; ECS: Extracellular fluid; CM: Cell membrane; ESL: Endothelial surface layer

Fig. 2.1. Distribution of body water across fluid compartments.

Table 2.1. Distribution of body water across fluid compartments as a percentage of body weight in dogs and cats.

	Dog	Cat
Total body water	60%	60%
Intracellular fluid	40%	40%
Extracellular fluid	20%	20%
Interstitial	14–16%	15–17%
Plasma volume	4–6%	3–5%
Blood volume	8–9%	5–7%

Table 2.2. Approximate distribution of electrolytes between the intracellular space (ICS) and extracellular space (ECS). These may vary depending on species and individual (Wellman *et al.*, 2012)

	ICS	ECS
Sodium	12	145
Potassium	140	4
Calcium	4	2.5
Magnesium	34	1
Chloride	4	110
Bicarbonate	12	24
Phosphates	40	2
Protein	50	7.5 (0–15)
Total osmolality	296	296

concentration of a solution) between the two compartments must be equal, otherwise a shift of water will occur. Normal osmolality in dogs and cats is reported to be 300 and 310 mOsm/kg, respectively (Hardy and Osborne, 1979; Chew *et al.*, 1991). This normal osmolality of the blood/body then sets the benchmark by which fluids are compared. A fluid is considered to be **hypotonic** if its osmolality is less than that of blood, **isotonic** if it is approximately equal, and **hypertonic** if it is greater.

In general, water always moves from an area of lower concentration to one of higher concentration. It is for this reason that osmolality is the major driving force for movement of fluid between the intracellular and extracellular space. For example, **hypotonic losses** (loss of water in excess of electrolytes) would cause a sudden increase in the extracellular sodium concentration (and thereby osmolality). This would establish a concentration gradient that would favor movement of water from the intracellular space (Fig. 2.2). The end result would be intracellular dehydration as well as the decrease in extracellular and total body water. Over time there will be an increase in intracellular osmolality through generation of idiogenic osmoles to allow return to more normal fluid balance between the compartments. Examples of hypotonic losses include evaporative losses across the respiratory tract and certain types of urinary losses.

It is important to note that **isotonic losses** (loss of water and electrolyte in equal parts compared with normal osmolality) will result in loss of fluid from the extracellular compartment, but will *not* result in a shift from the intracellular space. As there is no net change in extracellular osmolality with this type of loss, there will be no gradient for movement (Fig. 2.3). Isotonic losses are the most commonly experienced in a clinical setting (such as vomiting, diarrhea, or some urinary losses), and so this becomes important when anticipating volume replacement.

While uncommon, **hypertonic losses** (loss of electrolyte in excess of water) will result in a decrease in extracellular osmolality. As a result, there will be a net shift of water into the intracellular space down its concentration gradient (Fig. 2.4). Ultimately there will be a decrease in extracellular fluid and an increase in intracellular fluid, with a reduction in osmolality in both compartments. Over time there will be a reduction of intracellular osmolality to allow return to more normal fluid balance between the compartments. Examples of hypertonic losses include renal salt wasting, diuretic administration, and Addison's disease. There can also be circumstances whereby losses may be isotonic but are only replaced by water consumption and free water retention. This would also result in hyponatremia and effective hypertonic losses.

2.4 Movement between Intravascular and Interstitial Compartments

Movement of fluid, electrolytes, and proteins (colloids) between the intravascular and interstitial

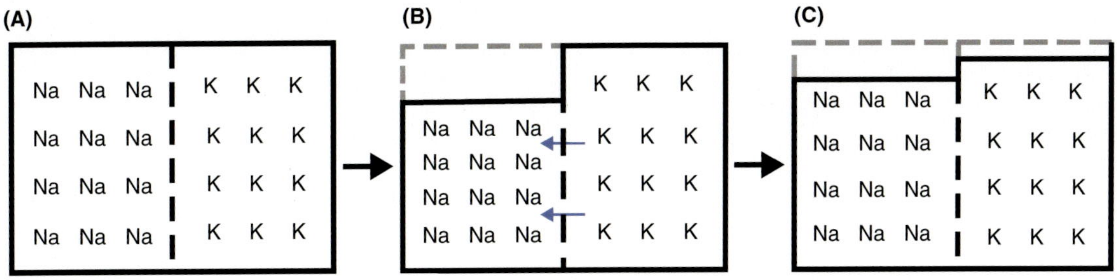

Fig. 2.2. Movement of water based on osmotic gradients: hypotonic loss. Schematic representation of an example fluid shift. (A) Normal electrolyte and water distribution. (B) Loss of free water from the extracellular compartment resulting in an increase in osmolality and a shift of water from the intracellular space (blue arrows). (C) Resulting change in fluid balance normalizing osmolality between the two compartments.

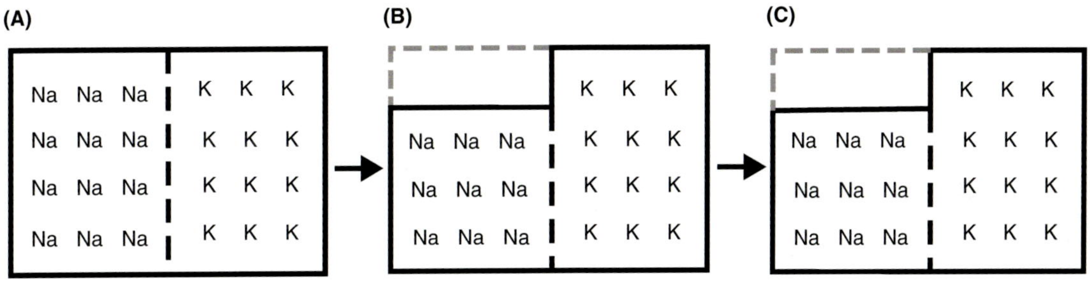

Fig. 2.3. Movement of water based on osmotic gradients: isotonic loss. Schematic representation of an example fluid shift. (A) Normal electrolyte and water distribution. (B) Loss of isotonic fluids results in no change in osmolality, so no shift of water occurs. (C) There will be no resulting change in intracellular fluid balance.

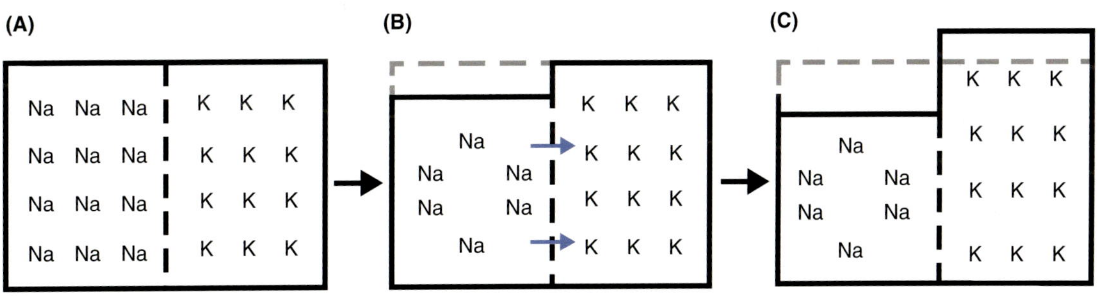

Fig. 2.4. Movement of water based on osmotic gradients: hypertonic loss. Schematic representation of an example fluid shift. (A) Normal electrolyte and water distribution. (B) Loss of hypertonic fluids from the extracellular compartment resulting in a decrease in osmolality and a shift of water into the intracellular space (blue arrows). (C) Resulting change in fluid balance normalizing osmolality between the two compartments.

spaces plays a major role in extracellular homeostasis. Therefore, the barrier function that exists between the two is essential to help regulate that movement and general fluid balance across the body. Further, as administered fluids must enter the vascular compartment for distribution, these relationships will have a huge impact on deciding fluid type and volume to administer. Water and electrolytes readily move between the vascular and interstitial spaces, and so osmotic forces do not play a major role as they do from intracellular and extracellular spaces. As such, traditionally the vascular endothelium and Starling's forces had been afforded credit for serving as the barrier and impacting fluid shifting. However, more recent evidence suggests that it is the delicate structure of the **endothelial surface layer** (ESL) that is the true gateway, particularly for protein trafficking and maintaining extracellular fluid balance. For perspective, a brief overview of the classic and revised view is presented below.

2.4.1 Classic view – Starling

For decades, the view of intravascular fluid regulation was dictated by the hypotheses put forward by Ernest Starling, which led to development of the Starling equation (Starling, 1896).

The Starling equation is based on the notion of forces which serve to push fluid into the opposing space (**hydrostatic**) or pull fluid back into the current space (**oncotic**). **Hydrostatic pressure** is the force exerted against the vascular wall either from the luminal side of the vessel (capillary hydrostatic pressure, or P_{cap}) or from the interstitial side (interstitial hydrostatic pressure, or P_{int}). **Oncotic pressure** is the portion of osmotic pressure exerted by proteins/macromolecules either within the vascular space (capillary oncotic pressure, or π_{cap}) or within the interstitium (interstitial oncotic pressure, or π_{int}). Osmotic pressure is dictated by the number of molecules, not the size. As there is a much great number of small molecules (electrolytes), proteins only contribute a fraction of overall osmotic pressure. However, given that electrolytes move freely across the endothelium and proteins do not move as readily, the only osmotic differential is therefore provided by these larger molecules. The other major component of the Starling equation relates to **endothelial permeability** (filtration coefficient, or K_f), and how readily macromolecules are able to move into the interstitium. This permeability was believed to be a function of the cleft or gap size in between endothelial cells. In turn, the size of these gaps could be affected by a number of factors, including tissue-specific differences based on function (e.g., low permeability in the glomerulus versus high permeability in the liver), or the impact of certain disease states (such as sepsis) (Boulpaep, 2009). The combination and balance of these different factors are then represented in the Starling equation and Fig. 2.5:

$$\text{Net filtration} = K_f\,(P_{cap} - P_{int}) - (\pi_{cap} - \pi_{int})$$

In this classic view proposed by Starling, there is a net loss of fluid to the interstitium on the arteriolar side of the capillary bed, the majority of which is reclaimed on the venous side (Table 2.3). This occurs because the P_{cap} is the predominant force in arteries, favoring movement out of the vascular space. However, as fluid moves into the interstitium, there is a decrease in P_{cap} such that, by the time it reaches venular circulation, π_{cap} is the predominant force shifting fluid back into the vascular space. Despite this, there is a net loss of fluid (approximately 5%) to the interstitium as blood moves across the capillary bed and into the venular system (Boulpaep, 2009). Making up the difference, and not represented in the Starling equation, is the important role that lymphatic drainage also plays in maintaining interstitial fluid balance. The associated increase in interstitial hydrostatic pressure promotes the movement of fluid into the lymphatic system to then be returned to systemic circulation (Boulpaep, 2009). There are a number of factors and disease processes that could serve to impact this delicate balance and potentially interstitial fluid balance. For example, hypoproteinemia would result in decreased π_{cap}, or congestive heart failure would cause increased P_{cap}, either of which could potentially lead to edema formation. The ability for changes in these

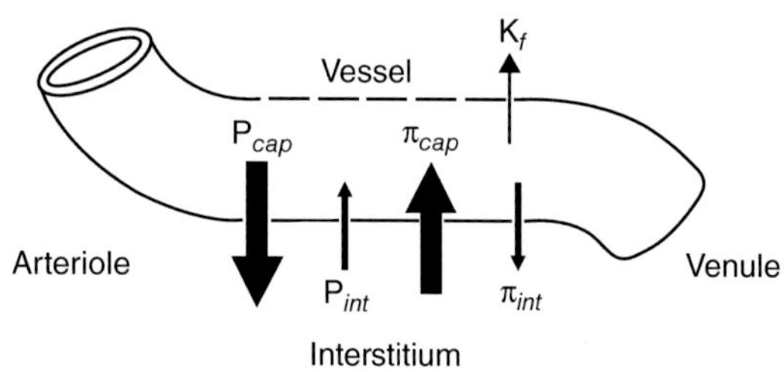

Fig. 2.5. Schematic representation of Starling's forces, and the relative impact on fluid shifts across the vessel wall. K_f, filtration coefficient; P_{cap}, capillary hydrostatic pressure; P_{int}, interstitial hydrostatic pressure; π_{cap}, capillary oncotic pressure; π_{int}, interstitial oncotic pressure. (© The Ohio State University.)

Table 2.3. Values for Starling forces in pre-capillary arterioles and post-capillary venules, along with net values. These are average values, with differences in specific tissue beds. All values in mm Hg (Boulpaep 2009).

	P_{cap}	P_{int}	π_{cap}	π_{int}	Net
Arteriolar end	+35	−2	+25	+0.1	+12
Venular end	+15	−2	+25	+3	−5

values to either increase or decrease the risk of edema formation is summarized in Table 2.4.

2.4.2 Revised view – Glycocalyx

While the precepts set by Starling have persisted, more recent recognition of the endothelial glycocalyx and its role in extracellular fluid balance has prompted some adjustment. The **glycocalyx** is formed by a collection of proteoglycan, glycoproteins, and glycosaminoglycans that cover the lumen surface of endothelial cells and serve to form the endothelial surface layer (Gaudette *et al.*, 2017). While an extensive review of the structure and function of the ESL is beyond the scope of this chapter, consideration of its impact is important in the context of the changing scope of fluid therapy. For those interested, there are comprehensive review articles available (Weinbaum *et al.*, 2007; Gaudette *et al.*, 2017).

The branching structure of the glycocalyx creates a lattice that incorporates plasma and soluble proteins such as albumin and fibronectin. Rather than the endothelial cells, this combination of components then conveys selectivity for the size (10–20 nm), shape, and charge (the ESL is negatively charged) of molecules that can pass between the vascular compartment and the interstitium (Gaudette *et al.*, 2017) (see Fig. 2.6 for a schematic representation). This is contrary to the previous notion that this function was the result of gaps between endothelial cells. The thickness and composition of the ESL can vary from one tissue bed to the next to allow selectivity of permeability (Gaudette *et al.*, 2017). Also contrary to what was proposed by Starling, it is the oncotic force within the space below the ESL (the **subglyceal space**), not the interstitium, that dictates the pressure gradient (Adamson *et al.*, 2004). This area is kept relatively free of proteins by a barrier created by albumin and other components of the ESL, as well as the rapid movement of fluid through the intra-endothelial cell clefts (Gaudette *et al.*, 2017). As a result, the oncotic gradient is much higher than it would be with the interstitium, thereby promoting vascular fluid retention. Further, this suggests that the movement of fluid between lumen to interstitium does not just occur at the ends of the capillary unit, but along the entire length (Adamson *et al.*, 2004). Another important difference is that the effect of the oncotic gradient serves to limit fluid loss to the interstitium, but does not promote overt reabsorption, as was previously believed (Adamson *et al.*, 2004).

With this understanding, the role of albumin becomes even more important. Not only does it contribute to the oncotic pressure gradient, but it also provides a lot of the charge barrier restricting the movement of macromolecules into the interstitium. Further, this revised view makes it clear how important the ESL is for normal fluid balance and endothelial function in health. It has also been shown that the ESL becomes affected in a number of diseases, particularly inflammatory processes like sepsis and trauma. The implications for fluid therapy are also incredibly important, as the ESL can impact distribution and effectiveness of administered fluids, and it can also be impacted by what type, how much and how quickly fluids are given.

2.5 Summary

Bringing together all these concepts, ultimately the goal is to understand what will happen to various

Table 2.4. Effect of changes in various factors impacting extracellular fluid balance on the risk of edema formation.

Force	Normal effect	Change	Risk of edema
Capillary oncotic	Pull fluid into intravascular space	↑ ↓	↓ ↑
Capillary hydrostatic	Push fluid into interstitial space	↑ ↓	↑ ↓
Interstitial oncotic	Pull fluid into interstitial space	↑ ↓	↑ ↓
Interstitial hydrostatic	Push fluid into intravascular space	↑ ↓	↓ ↑
Filtration coefficient	Increase movement into the interstitium	↑ ↓	↑ ↓
Lymphatic drainage	Clear net loss of fluid to interstitial space	↑ ↓	↓ ↑

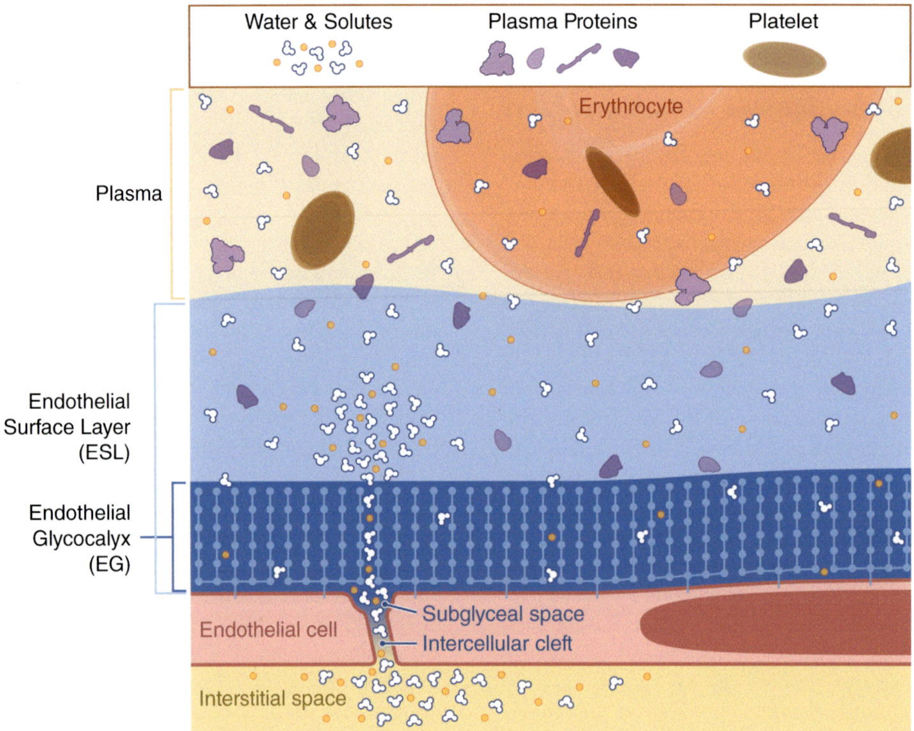

Fig. 2.6. Schematic representation of the glycocalyx and endothelial surface layer. (© The Ohio State University.)

constituents of fluids when they are administered. This, in turn, will impact fluid choice and volume to be administered. Free water (hypotonic fluid) can move across all body fluid compartments based on concentration gradients (**distribution of free water = total body water**). Given their small size, administered electrolytes can move freely across the endothelium/ESL, but cannot move across the cell membrane without active transport (**distribution of electrolytes = extracellular space**). Large molecules like proteins (colloids) are relatively restricted from moving into the interstitium by the ESL, at least initially and/or in healthy states (**distribution of colloids = vascular space**).

With this framework, the next two chapters will provide an overview of the different types of fluids available, and the clinical circumstances for which they may be used.

References

Adamson, R.H., Lenz, J.F., Zhang, X. *et al.* (2004) Oncotic pressures opposing filtration across non-fenestrated rat microvessels. *Journal of Physiology* 557, 889–907.

Boulpaep, E. (2009) The Microcirculation. In: Boron, W.F. and Boulpaep, E.L. (eds) *Medical Physiology*, 1st edn. Saunders Elsevier, Philadelphia, pp. 463–482.

Chew, D.J., Leonard, M. and Muir, W.W. (1991) Effect of sodium bicarbonate infusion on serum osmolality, electrolyte concentrations and blood gas tensions in cats. *American Journal of Veterinary Research* 52, 12–18.

Gaudette, S., Hughes, D. and Boller, M. (2017) The endothelial glycocalyx: structure and function in health and critical illness. *Journal of Veterinary Emergency and Critical Care* 30, 117–134.

Hardy, R.M. and Osborne, C.A. (1979) Water deprivation test in the dog: maximal normal values. *Journal of the American Veterinary Medical Association* 174, 479–489.

Jain, N.C. (1986) *Schalm's Veterinary Hematology*. Lea & Febiger, Philadelphia.

Kohn, K. and DiBartola, S. (2000) Composition and distribution of body fluids in dogs and cats. In: DiBartola, S. (ed.) *Fluid Therapy in Small Animal Practice*, 2nd edn. W.B. Saunders, Philadelphia, pp. 6–27.

MacIntire, D.K. (2008) Pediatric fluid therapy. *Veterinary Clinics of North America Small Animal Practice* 38, 621–627.

Stanton C.A., Hamar, D.W., Johnson, D.E. *et al.* (1992) Bioelectrical impedance and zoometry for body composition analysis in domestic cats. *American Journal of Veterinary Research* 53, 251–259.

Starling, E.H. (1896) On the absorption of fluids from the connective tissue spaces. *Journal of Physiology* 19, 312–326.

Wamberg, S., Sandgaard, N.C.F. and Bie, P. (2002) Simultaneous determination of total body water and plasma volume in conscious dogs by the indicator dilution principle. *Journal of Nutrition* 132, 1171S.

Weinbaum, S., Tarbell, J.M. and Damiano, E.R. (2007) The structure and function of the endothelial glycocalyx layer. *The Annual Review of Biomedical Engineering* 9, 121–167.

Wellman, M.L., DiBartola, S. and Kohn, C.W. (2012) Applied physiology of body fluids in dogs and cats. In: DiBartola, S. (ed.) *Fluid, Electrolyte and Acid–Base Disorders in Small Animal Practice*, 4th edn. W.B. Saunders, Philadelphia, pp. 2–25.

3 Fluid Types – Crystalloids

Edward Cooper

The Ohio State University, Columbus, Ohio, USA

The next step on the fluid therapy journey is consideration of the various types of fluids, and how their properties might impact decision making. Despite extensive investigation, no one type of fluid is ideal for every clinical scenario, as they all have potential benefits and drawbacks. Careful consideration of the goals for administering fluids is therefore needed to best tailor to the individual patient. This chapter will focus specifically on **crystalloids**, which are solutions with varying electrolyte compositions in water (whereas the next chapter will focus on colloids). Crystalloids are primarily classified based on their tonicity (or osmolarity). As discussed in Chapter 2, osmolality is the same across body fluid compartments and is the reference point for comparing fluids. Recognizing that there will be analyzer differences, Table 3.1 presents a composite of approximate electrolytes' values and osmolality for dogs and cats. This will serve as a reference point when comparing fluid composition to "normal" patient values. Fluids that have a lower osmolarity than normal are considered **hypotonic**, those with an approximately equal osmolarity are **isotonic**, and those with a higher osmolarity are considered **hypertonic**. Crystalloids can be further classified based on their effects on acid–base balance, as some can be acidifying while others are more alkalinizing. Ideally the type of crystalloid used should match what is needed based on what has been lost and/or needs to be replaced/provided. Careful consideration of their various characteristics, potential applications, and contraindications should help in that process.

3.1 Hypotonic Crystalloids

3.1.1 Composition

By definition, hypotonic fluids have an osmolarity (tonicity) that is lower than that of blood, implying that they provide water in excess of electrolytes. Because of this, the volume of distribution for hypotonic fluids is the total body water. When administered, the resulting decrease in osmolarity of the extracellular space will create an osmotic gradient for the movement of water into the intracellular space. Examples of hypotonic fluids are shown in Fig. 3.1 and their respective compositions can be found in Table 3.2. When comparing with Table 3.1, it is clear these have much lower electrolyte concentrations compared with normal blood. It is important to note, however, that the reported osmolarity of 5% dextrose in water (D5W) and 0.45% NaCl + 2.5% dextrose is similar to that of normal blood. This raises the question as to why these fluids are considered hypotonic, rather than isotonic. Largely this is due to a concept called **effective osmolarity**. After administration of these fluids, there is relatively rapid intracellular movement and metabolism of the dextrose. As a result, the water and electrolytes left behind are what reflect the effective osmolarity. For example, the osmolarity of D5W as a solution is 252 mOsm/kg, but the effective osmolarity is 0 as it contains no electrolytes (see Table 3.2). Dextrose has been added to these fluids so that as they are administered there is less of an osmolarity difference that could result in osmotic injury to red blood cells or endothelium. However, unless delivered rapidly, even solutions with a lower osmolarity (such as 0.45% NaCl or Normosol M) can be safely administered.

3.1.2 Indications for use

As hypotonic fluids have a lower sodium content relative to water, they are ideally suited to replacement of a free water deficit. A free water deficit is typically reflected by the presence of hypernatremia, and careful correction is needed to avoid changing the sodium too quickly. Specific guidelines for management of these patients is provided in Chapter 8vi (Management of Hypernatremia

DOI: 10.1079/9781789243406.0003

Table 3.1. Approximate electrolytes' values and osmolarity in dogs and cats. (All values in mEq/l except osmolarity, which is in mOsm/l.)

Species	Sodium	Potassium	Chloride	Ionized calcium	Ionized magnesium	Osmolarity
Dog	135–145	4–5	110	2.4–3	2.4	280–305
Cat	140–155	4–5	120	2.2–2.8	2.1	295–320

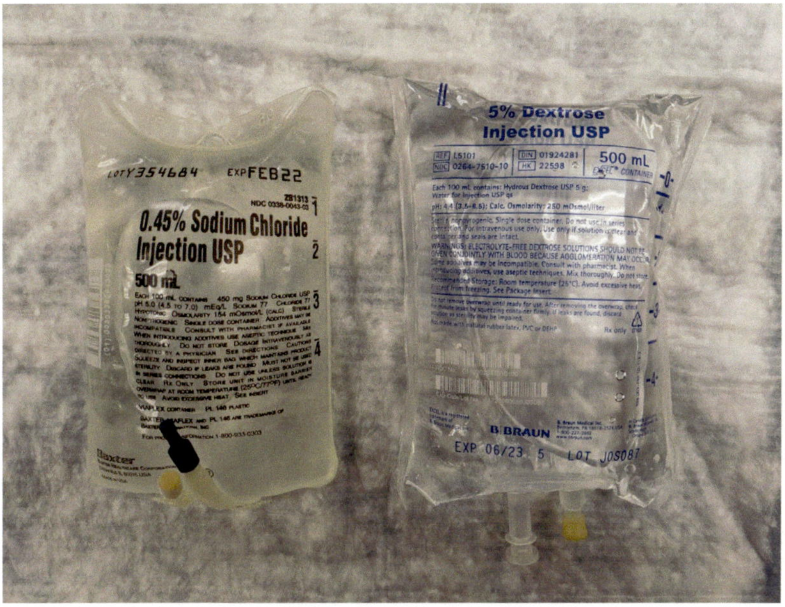

Fig. 3.1. Examples of hypotonic fluids: 0.45% NaCl and 5% dextrose in water.

Table 3.2. Composition of available hypotonic fluids. (All values in mEq/l except osmolarity, which is in mOsm/l.)

Fluid	Sodium	Potassium	Chloride	Ionized Ca	Ionized Mg	Osmolarity	Effective osmolarity	Bicarb precursor
5% Dextrose	0	0	0	0	0	252	0	n/a
0.45% NaCl	77	0	77	0	0	154	154	n/a
0.45% NaCl + 2.5% dextrose	77	0	77	0	0	280	154	n/a
Normosol M	40	13	40	0	3	100	100	Acetate

and Hyponatremia). Patients with kidney disease and/or cardiac disease have a significantly reduced tolerance for sodium load. Use of a hypotonic fluid in these patients can help decrease the risk of fluid overload and prevent the exacerbation of clinical conditions that could come from administration of fluids containing more sodium. See Chapter 8iii (Impact of Cardiac Disease on Fluid Therapy) and Chapter 8iv (Impact of Renal Disease on Fluid Therapy) for more information about fluid therapy in these patients. Finally, daily physiologic fluid needs are generally more water than sodium. As such, hypotonic fluids are better suited to provision of "maintenance" fluid therapy compared with other fluid types. Chapter 6iii (Maintenance Fluid Therapy) provides additional information on the use of hypotonic fluids for this purpose.

3.1.3 Contraindications and adverse effects

While hypotonic fluids may have many applications, they are least suited for use in fluid resuscitation. As described in Chapter 6i, the goal of resuscitation is expansion of the vascular volume to support the cardiovascular system. However, as mentioned above, hypotonic fluids distribute across the total body water. This means only a small portion will remain in the vascular space after redistribution. As such, they will not be very effective in this role unless a very large volume is administered. Further, rapid administration of hypotonic fluids could be harmful by causing sudden changes in blood osmolarity. This, in turn, could result in osmotic injury secondary to the associated shift of water into the intracellular space. Of greatest importance would be the potential to cause red blood cell lysis, damage to vascular endothelium, or neuronal edema and disruption of the central nervous system. For all these reasons, hypotonic fluids should *not* be used for fluid resuscitation.

In addition to these concerns, there are other potential adverse effects that could be associated with administration of hypotonic fluids. If used to replace isotonic losses (dehydration without hypernatremia) or address hypovolemia, there is potential to cause hyponatremia. This occurs because water is being replaced in excess of sodium, and dehydrated patients are often in a very water-retentive state (increased release of anti-diuretic hormone). In fact, several studies in sick human adults and pediatric patients have shown an increased incidence of hyponatremia even when used for maintenance purposes (Foster *et al.*, 2014; Okada *et al.*, 2017). In veterinary medicine, use of hypotonic fluids for true maintenance needs is still recommended, with risk of hyponatremia being low unless the patient is hypovolemic (Hansen and Vigani, 2017). Another potential adverse effect of hypotonic fluids which contain dextrose is the risk of causing hyperglycemia. This is unlikely in healthy patients with a normally functioning pancreas, as the normal mechanism for maintaining glycemic control will be intact. However, this may be a limiting factor for use of these fluids in patients with diabetes mellitus. Further, the stress response and associated insulin resistance in critically ill patients may impact glucose regulation and increase the risk of developing hyperglycemia (Knieriem *et al.*, 2007; Yamada *et al.*, 2017).

3.2 Isotonic Crystalloids

3.2.1 Composition

As previously stated, isotonic crystalloids have an osmolarity similar to that of blood. As a result, administration of these fluids will not cause a significant change in osmolarity, and so will be distributed across the extracellular space. With this in mind, the electrolyte composition is targeted to match that compartment (predominantly sodium and chloride), though there is some variability among the different available fluids (Table 3.3). Examples are shown in Fig. 3.2. This variability allows isotonic crystalloids to be further categorized based on their comparison to blood electrolyte distribution. **"Normal" saline** (0.9% NaCl) contains only equal amounts of sodium and chloride (each at 154 mEq/l) with no other electrolytes. In comparison with the normal values presented in Table 3.1, overall this fluid is not well matched. On the other hand, the **balanced electrolyte solutions** (lactated Ringer's solution, Plasma-Lyte A, and Normosol R) contain concentrations of sodium and chloride that more closely match those found in blood, as well as additional electrolytes (potassium and calcium or magnesium). This would suggest potential advantage of these fluids over 0.9% NaCl (see indications for use below).

Isotonic crystalloids can also have impacts on acid–base balance. Owing to its high chloride content compared with blood, normal saline has an acidifying effect. Essentially, it causes a disproportionate increase in the patient's chloride relative to sodium. As a result, there is a decrease in bicarbonate (to maintain electroneutrality) and associated

Table 3.3. Composition of available isotonic fluids. (All values in mEq/l, except osmolarity, which is in mOsm/l.)

Fluid	Sodium	Potassium	Chloride	Ionized Ca	Ionized Mg	Osmolarity	Bicarb precursor
0.9% NaCl	154	0	154	0	0	308	n/a
Lactated Ringer's	130	4	109	3	0	278	Lactate
Normosol R	140	5	98	0	3	294	Gluconate and acetate
Plasma-Lyte A	140	5	98	0	3	294	

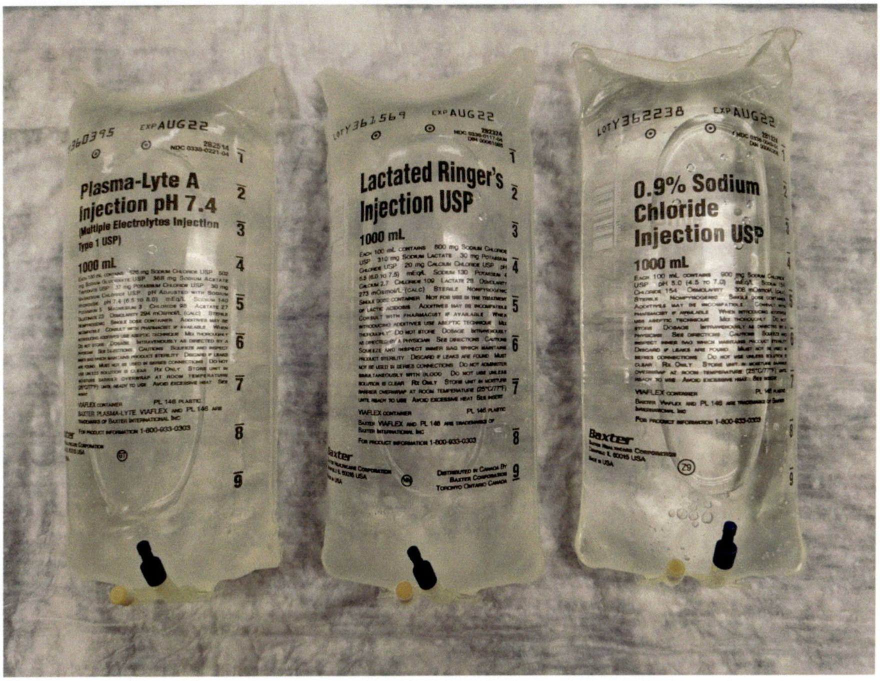

Fig. 3.2. Examples of isotonic fluids: Plasma-Lyte A, lactated Ringer's, and 0.9% NaCl.

metabolic acidosis. The balanced electrolyte solutions, on the other hand, have more of an alkalinizing effect through mechanisms that vary depending on the solution. For Normosol and Plasma-Lyte, they have a decrease in chloride relative to sodium which promotes bicarbonate retention. In addition, the balanced electrolyte solutions contain precursors that lead to the generation of bicarbonate and thereby have a buffering/alkalinizing effect. The lactate in lactated Ringer's solution can also promote the consumption of hydrogen ions to reduce acidosis. The mechanisms for these are summarized in Box 3.1.

Box 3.1. Mechanisms.

Normosol R and Plasma-Lyte

Acetate:

$$NaC_2H_3O_2 + 2O_2 \rightarrow CO_2 + H_2O + NaHCO_3\text{-}$$

Gluconate:

$$NaC_6H_{11}O_2 + 5\,½O_2 \rightarrow 5CO_2 + 5H_2O + NaHCO_3\text{-}$$

Lactated Ringer's solution

Lactate:

$$NaC_3H_5O_3 + 3O_2 \rightarrow 2CO_2 + 2H_2O + NaHCO_3\text{-}$$
$$2C_3H_5O_3 + 2H^+ \rightarrow C_6H_{12}O_6 \text{ (gluconeogenesis)}$$
$$C_3H_5O_3 + H^+ + 3O_2 \rightarrow 3CO_2 + 3H_2O$$

3.2.2 Indications for use

Isotonic crystalloids are the most widely used and versatile type of fluid, having a variety of applications. As such, they can be utilized in all phases of fluid therapy. Isotonic fluids have been shown to be effective in resuscitation. Their isotonic nature allows for rapid administration without risk of osmotic injury. While they redistribute across the extracellular compartment, sufficient administration will allow for expansion of vascular volume to support the cardiovascular system. See Chapter 6i for more information and recommendations regarding their use in resuscitation. As most losses are isotonic in nature, these fluids also lend themselves well to replacement of dehydration and ongoing losses. Use of isotonic fluid for replacement fluid therapy is described in Chapter 6ii. However, concurrent hypernatremia would suggest free water loss and a hypotonic fluid would be more beneficial. Further, isotonic fluids are often used to provide maintenance fluid requirements. Recognizing that true maintenance requirement is better matched with a hypotonic fluid (Hansen and Vigani, 2017), for many practitioners use of an isotonic fluid serves to simplify the process through the use of only one type of fluid. While this results in more sodium administration than needed, the patient will excrete the excess without negative impact. Notable exceptions to this would be patients with either cardiac or renal disease (Hansen and Vigani, 2017).

The potential to impact acid–base balance yields additional applications for isotonic crystalloids. The alkalinizing effects of the balanced electrolyte solutions could have some benefit for patients with a **metabolic acidosis** (e.g., increased lactate in shock, diabetic ketoacidosis, renal disease). Patients with **metabolic alkalosis** secondary to a low chloride (such as vomiting from a high gastrointestinal obstruction) would potentially benefit from administration of 0.9% NaCl. The high chloride content in that fluid would allow for the most rapid correction of that disturbance. In addition, the high sodium and chloride content of 0.9% NaCl promotes calcium excretion through the kidneys, making it the fluid of choice for hypercalcemic patients.

3.2.3 Contraindications and adverse effects

As previously mentioned, isotonic crystalloids will redistribute across the extracellular compartment, with a significant portion ending up in the interstitium (classically two-thirds to three-quarters of the administered volume). In circumstances of interstitial dehydration, this would be of benefit. However, if the goal is to replace acute loss from the intravascular space (volume resuscitation), then the addition of significant fluid to the interstitium could result in tissue edema. In general, excessive volume administration (volume overload), particularly in the face of kidney or cardiac disease, could also result in tissue edema. For this reason, there should be caution in the use of isotonic crystalloids for these patients that are less tolerant of sodium load. The associated accumulation of fluid in the pulmonary interstitium, gastrointestinal track, peripheral tissues, etc., could potentially be associated with significant adverse consequences (Cotton *et al.*, 2006). See Chapter 6i for more descriptions of this in the context of fluid resuscitation.

There are several potential adverse effects associated with administration of isotonic crystalloids. As noted, isotonic crystalloids can help in the correction of acid–base disturbances, and along similar lines could be responsible for creating them. Most notable is the potential for 0.9% NaCl to create or contribute to metabolic acidosis. As 0.9% NaCl is equal parts sodium and chloride, the patient is receiving excess chloride compared with normal blood (154 mEq/l compared with about 110 mEq/l). The resulting hyperchloremia will cause a reduction in bicarbonate and associated metabolic acidosis. For this reason, 0.9% NaCl should be avoided in patients with an existing acidemia.

In addition to the potential effects on acid–base balance, 0.9% NaCl has also been implicated as a potential cause of acute kidney injury, particularly in critically ill patients (Shaw *et al.*, 2014; Yunos *et al.*, 2015). While the mechanisms are not entirely understood, it is thought to be related to the increased filtration and delivery of chloride through the nephron. Higher concentrations of chloride to the macula densa (where the distal convoluted tubule passes by the glomerulus) can trigger vasoconstriction of the afferent arteriole. The result is a decrease in renal blood flow and glomerular filtration rate. This is part of the mechanism known as **tubuloglomerular feedback** (Rose and Post, 2001). Patients with severe dehydration, hypovolemia or existing kidney disease may be at increased risk of this adverse effect (Glassford and Bellomo, 2018). While the implications of this have not yet been determined in veterinary medicine, caution should be used with application of 0.9% NaCl in these circumstances.

3.3 Hypertonic Crystalloids

3.3.1 Composition

Hypertonic solutions have an osmolarity that exceeds normal blood osmolality. Most often this entails the use of **hypertonic saline** (HTS) ranging from a 3% to 7% NaCl solution as administered (see Table 3.4). It is important to note that HTS also comes as a 23.4% solution (Fig. 3.3). However, this is too concentrated and *must* be diluted before administration, to avoid severe phlebitis/vascular injury. This can be accomplished by diluting the 23.4% HTS with sterile water or 0.9% NaCl. See Clinical Case 3.1 at the end of this chapter for an example of how to perform this dilution. Mannitol

Table 3.4. Composition of available hypertonic fluids. (All values in mEq/l except osmolarity, which is in mOsm/l.)

Fluid	Sodium	Potassium	Chloride	Ionized Ca	Ionized Mg	Osmolarity	Bicarb precursor
3% NaCl	513	0	513	0	0	1026	n/a
7% NaCl	1198	0	1198	0	0	2396	n/a
23.4% NaCl	4000	0	4000	0	0	8000	
20% Mannitol	0	0	0	0	0	1372	

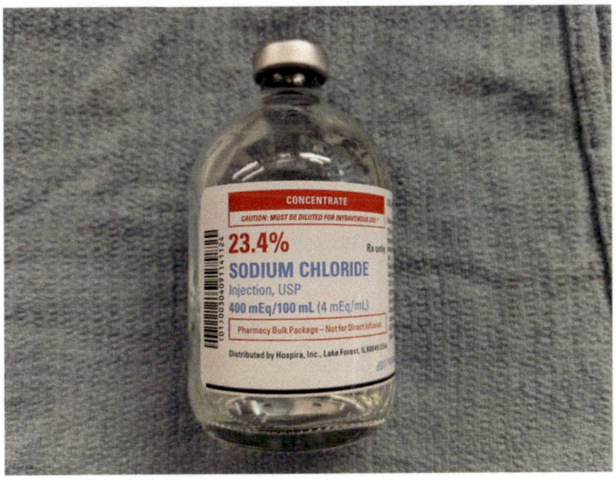

Fig. 3.3. A bottle of 23.4% NaCl. Note that this concentration must always be diluted to 7–7.5% prior to administration.

is also considered a hypertonic fluid, with an osmolarity comparable to 4% NaCl.

With intravenous administration, the initial effect of hypertonic fluids will be to draw fluid into the vascular space. As a result, there will be an increase in circulating volume in excess of the amount administered. While this has been reported to be as much as 3–5× the amount given, it has been shown that the effect may be much less than that (only about 1.2×) (Silverstein *et al.*, 2005). It is also important to note that this volume expansion will be short-lived, as the fluid and electrolytes will redistribute across the extracellular space within 30–60 min.

3.3.2 Indications for use

Given the potential to promote acute expansion of the vascular volume, hypertonic fluids can be used in **resuscitation**. These fluids potentially carry the benefit of only having to administer a relatively small amount compared with isotonic fluids. For this purpose, HTS (most often 7%) would be used over mannitol, as the latter would ultimately result in volume loss through osmotic diuresis. Hypertonic saline does not promote diuresis, as hypovolemia will trigger mechanisms for sodium and water retention. See Chapter 6i for more information regarding the use of HTS in resuscitation. It is important to mention that while HTS may be helpful in the resuscitation phase of fluid therapy, the effects will be short-lived as volume redistributes across the extracellular space. In this regard, HTS should be reserved for circumstances of severe hypovolemia and impending cardiovascular collapse. Further, it will typically be necessary to concurrently administer other types of resuscitative fluids.

Another major application of hypertonic fluids is in the treatment of cerebral edema and increased intracranial pressure (ICP), such as occurs with **traumatic brain injury**. As previously indicated, hypertonic fluids will result in the movement of fluid from the interstitium into the vascular space by increasing blood osmolality. While the fluid and electrolytes will ultimately redistribute back across the extracellular space, the blood–brain barrier will prevent that movement into the cerebral interstitium. This net effect is a decrease in brain volume and a reduction of ICP. Both HTS and mannitol can be used for this purpose, each carrying potential benefits and drawbacks (Pigott and Rudloff, 2021). They are equivalent in their ability to reduce intracranial pressure, but HTS carries the added benefit of volume expansion and blood pressure support compared with mannitol (Pigott and Rudloff, 2021). For this reason, HTS would be preferred in patients with a concurrent increase in ICP and hypovolemia-induced hypotension.

Patients experiencing acute **hyponatremia** may also benefit from administration of hypertonic saline, particularly if neurological signs have resulted. The concentration of NaCl used, as well as the rate of delivery, needs to be carefully selected based on the desired change in serum sodium. See Chapter 8vi for more information regarding sodium correction.

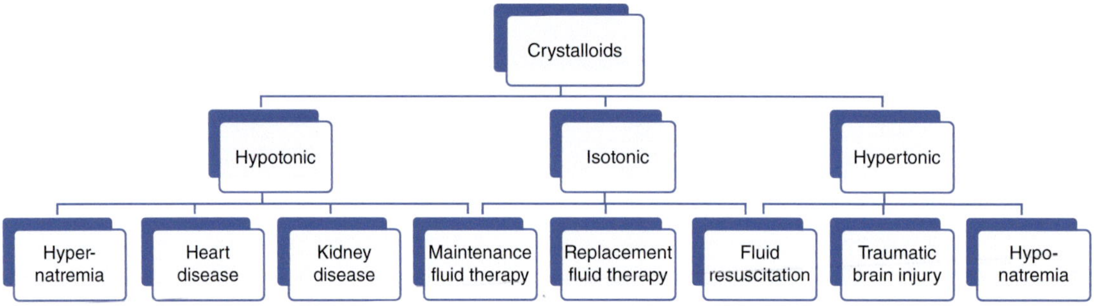

Fig. 3.4. Suggested applications of hypotonic, isotonic, and hypertonic crystalloids.

Clinical Case 3.1

You are presented with a 10 kg canine patient approximately 30 min after the patient has been hit by a car. On initial assessment the patient is exhibiting signs of shock and altered mentation with evidence of head trauma. You are concerned about hypotension and traumatic brain injury so you decide to give 7% HTS at 4 ml/kg over 5 min (see Chapter 6i for more information on why this was chosen). As you have a 23.4% NaCl stock solution, this will need to be diluted with sterile water.

The best approach to calculating dilutions is to use $V_1 \times C_1 = V_2 \times C_2$ where:

V_1 = volume of stock solution – ?
C_1 = concentration of stock solution – 23.4%
V_2 = final desired volume – 40 ml (4 ml/kg × 10 kg)
C_2 = final desired concentration – 7%

The volume of 23.4% NaCl needed is the only unknown, so the equation is rearranged:

$$V_1 = (V_2 \times C_2) / C_1 = (40 \text{ ml} \times 7\%) / 23.4\% = 12 \text{ ml}$$

As the target volume is 40 ml, 12 ml of 23.4% NaCl added to 28 ml of sterile water will result in a 7% NaCl solution.

If sterile water is not available, 0.9% NaCl could also be used to dilute the 23.4%, though a slight adjustment of the calculation would be needed. To account for the presence of 0.9%, the target concentration is set at 6.1% instead of 7%:

$$V_1 = (V_2 \times C_2) / C_1 = (40 \text{ ml} \times 6.1\%) / 23.4\% = 10.4 \text{ ml}$$

As the target volume is 40 ml, 10.4 ml of 23.4% NaCl added to 29.6 ml of 0.9% NaCl will result in a 7% NaCl solution.

3.3.3 Contraindications and adverse effects

Dehydration is considered a relative contraindication to use of hypertonic fluids. This makes some sense, given that the goal of these fluids is to pull fluid from the extravascular space. A dehydrated patient has a decrease in interstitial fluid, and so HTS might not be as effective at expanding the vascular volume in that regard. However, even with significant dehydration, osmosis is osmosis, and water will still move down its concentration gradient. It has been shown that use of HTS in dehydrated animals resulted in similar efficacy and no adverse effects when compared with normally hydrated subjects (Wade *et al.*, 1992). Further argument against using HTS in dehydration is that it may serve to worsen the interstitial deficit. However, as previously stated, any fluid that moves from interstitium to vascular compartment will redistribute after 30–60 min, making the net loss of fluid negligible.

Another potential concern with regard to the use of HTS is the potential to trigger a reflex **bradycardia** if administered too quickly. This can come about as rapid volume expansion that triggers atrial stretch receptors, resulting in increased vagal tone. Acute hyperosmolality can also trigger **vasodilation**, and potentially cause a transient decrease in blood pressure. While these effects are short-lived, it is recommended not to administer HTS any faster than 0.5–1.0 ml/kg/min. In addition, rapid volume expansion could have adverse effects in the actively bleeding patient by promoting further blood loss through increased pressure and disruption of blood clots. See Chapter 8i for more information regarding fluid administration in the hemorrhaging patient. Hypertonic fluids should also be avoided in patients with a low tolerance for sodium load, such as those with cardiac or kidney disease.

3.4 Summary

The decision regarding which type of crystalloid to use should be based on the goal of fluid administration, as well as the respective properties and consideration of potential adverse effects. Figure 3.4 depicts an overall summary of the most common applications of crystalloid solutions.

References

Cotton, B.A., Guy, J.S., Morris, J.A. *et al.* (2006) The cellular, metabolic, and systemic consequences of aggressive fluid resuscitation strategies. *Shock* 26(2), 115–121.

Foster, B.A., Tom, D. and Hill, V. (2014) Hypotonic versus isotonic fluids in hospitalized children: a systematic review and meta-analysis. *The Journal of Pediatrics* 165(1), 163–169.

Glassford, N.J. and Bellomo, R. (2018) Does fluid type and amount affect kidney function in critical illness? *Critical Care Clinics* 34(2), 279–298.

Hansen, B. and Vigani, A. (2017) Maintenance fluid therapy: isotonic versus hypotonic solutions. *Veterinary Clinics of North America Small Animal Practice* 47(2), 383–395.

Knieriem, M., Otto, C.M. and Macintire, D. (2007) Hyperglycemia in critically ill patients. *Compendium of Continuing Education for Veterinarians* 29(6), 364–372.

Okada, M., Egi, M., Yokota, Y. *et al.* (2017) Comparison of the incidences of hyponatremia in adult postoperative critically ill patients receiving intravenous maintenance fluids with 140 mmol/L or 35 mmol/L of sodium: retrospective before/after observational study. *Journal of Anesthesia* 31(5), 657–663.

Pigott, A. and Rudloff, E. (2021) Traumatic brain injury – a review of intravenous therapy. *Frontiers in Veterinary Science* 8, 643800.

Rose, B.D. and Post, T.W. (2001) Renal circulation and glomerular filtration rate. In: Rose, B.D. and Post, T.W. (eds) *Clinical Physiology of Acid-Base and Electrolyte Disorders*. Mcgraw-Hill, New York, pp. 42–46.

Shaw, A.D., Raghunathan, K., Peyerl, F.W. *et al.* (2014) Association between intravenous chloride load during resuscitation and in-hospital mortality among patients with SIRS. *Intensive Care Medicine* 40(12), 1897–1905.

Silverstein, D.C., Aldrich, J., Haskins, S.C. *et al.* (2005) Assessment of changes in blood volume in response to resuscitative fluid administration in dogs. *Journal of Veterinary Emergency and Critical Care* 15(3), 185–192.

Wade, C.E., Tillman, F.J., Loveday, J.A. *et al.* (1992) Effect of dehydration on cardiovascular responses and electrolytes after hypertonic saline/dextran treatment for moderate hemorrhage. *Annals of Emergency Medicine* 21(2), 113–119.

Yamada, T., Shojima, N., Noma, H. *et al.* (2017) Glycemic control, mortality, and hypoglycemia in critically ill patients: a systematic review and network meta-analysis of randomized controlled trials. *Intensive Care Medicine*, 43(1), 1–15.

Yunos, N.M., Bellomo, R., Glassford, N. *et al.* (2015) Chloride-liberal vs. chloride-restrictive intravenous fluid administration and acute kidney injury: an extended analysis. *Intensive Care Medicine* 41(2), 257–264.

4i Synthetic Colloids

ANDA YOUNG

The Ohio State University, Columbus, Ohio, USA

In addition to the crystalloid solutions discussed in the previous chapter, the other major category of fluids for consideration is colloids. A colloid solution typically contains macromolecules (> 10 kDA) suspended in crystalloid solution. As these larger molecules tend to remain within the vascular space, they have the ability to transiently increase **intravascular oncotic pressure** (π_c), also known as **colloid osmotic pressure** (COP). Their overall ability to impact COP relies on the number of particles maintained within the vasculature (rather than the size), as well as the overall permeability of the endothelial surface layer (see Chapter 2 for additional information) (Grimm *et al.*, 2015; Casey *et al.*, 2018). Colloidal solutions can be classified as **natural** or **synthetic.** Chapter 4i will focus primarily on synthetic colloids, with Chapter 4ii focused on the natural colloids.

4i.1 Synthetic Colloidal Solutions

In health, COP is maintained predominantly by albumin, which supports intravascular volume in concert with the endothelial glycocalyx via its large molecular size (69 kDa), negative charge, and ability to attract sodium and water (Gibbs-Donnan effect). In addition to maintenance of COP, albumin participates in drug carriage and detoxification, binding of nitric oxide, and regulation of inflammation (Rozga *et al.*, 2013; Casey *et al.*, 2018). As such, albumin is considered the reference, or "natural" colloid. Despite these benefits, the associated costs and limited availability of albumin-containing products in certain regions prompted the development of semi-synthetic colloids. Similar resource limitations plague veterinary medicine to an even greater extent. Additionally, the administration of HSA to canine patients may result in delayed type III hypersensitivity reactions due to incomplete protein homology (Cazzolli and Prittie, 2015). As such, semi-synthetic colloids offer the benefit of being a cost-effective and readily available resource for volume expansion. An understanding of composition and application of semi-synthetic colloids allows for better consideration of the potential benefits and risks that are associated with their use.

Synthetic colloids generally come in three varieties: **dextrans** (linear glucose polymers), **gelatins** (bovine collagen derivatives), and **starches** (branched glucose polymers) (Casey *et al.*, 2018). Unique properties of select colloids are detailed in Table 4i.1.

4i.1.1 Dextrans

Dextrans are a class of volume expanders consisting of glucose polymers synthesized from the fermentation of sucrose via the bacterium *Leuconostoc mesenteroides* (Wong and Koenig, 2017). Dextrans are composed of polydisperse molecules with molecular weights ranging from 40 kDa (e.g., Dextran-40) to 70 kDa (e.g., Dextran-70) often suspended in D5W or 0.9% NaCl (Drobatz *et al.*, 2019). The individual properties of dextran solutions have resulted in a unique adverse event profile including anaphylaxis, bleeding tendencies, osmotic nephrosis and **acute kidney injury** (AKI) (Joannidis *et al.*, 2017; Brown and Semler, 2019). Additionally, Dextran-70 has antithrombotic effects that may be attributed to dilution of coagulation factors, decreased activity of vWF and FVIII, and disturbed fibrin polymerization and stability (Schott *et al.*, 2018). These findings support a significant role of a general colloidal dilutional coagulopathy. Although judicious dosing of dextrans may reduce the effects on coagulation, risk of AKI secondary to hyperoncotic impairment of glomerular filtration and osmotic tubular damage continues to limit their use (Joannidis *et al.*, 2017).

DOI: 10.1079/9781789243406.00041

Table 4i.1. Properties of select available synthetic colloid solutions.

Colloid	Conc.	Carrier fluid	MW (kDa)	Molar substitution	C2:C6 ratio	COP (mmHg)	Maximum daily dose (ml/kg/day)
Dextran							
Dextran-70	6%	0.9% NaCl	70	NA	NA	62	15–20
Gelatin							
Succinylated fluid gelatin	4%	0.9% NaCl	30	NA	NA	34	Unspecified
Urea cross-linked gelatin	3.5%	0.9% NaCl	35	NA	NA	15	Unspecified
Hetastarch							
Hespan	6%	0.9% NaCl	600	0.75	4–5:1	26	20
Hextend	6%	LRS	670	0.75	4:1	31	20
Pentastarch							
Pentaspan	10%	0.9% NaCl	200	0.4–0.5	4–5:1	66	30
Tetrastarch							
Voluven	10%	0.9% NaCl	130	0.38–0.45	9:1	70–80	50
Voluven	6%	0.9% NaCl	130	0.38–0.45	9:1	36	50
Vetstarch	6%	0.9% Nacl	130	0.38–0.45	9:1	36	50

Data from Holowaychuk, M.K. (2019) Colloid Fluid Therapy. In: Drobatz, K.J., Hopper, K., Rozanski, E.A. and Silverstein, D.C. (eds) *Textbook of Small Animal Emergency Medicine*, 1st edn. Wiley, Hoboken, New Jersey, Chapter 169, p. 1097.

4i.1.2 Gelatins

Gelatins are a class of volume expanders derived from the hydrolysis of bovine collagen. Gelatins are composed of polydisperse molecules, but the majority of molecules are <30 kDa (Drobatz *et al.*, 2019). The adverse event profile of gelatins includes allergic reactions and AKI. Additional risk of prion transmission, histamine release and coagulopathy has led to recommendations against their use for fluid resuscitation (Joannidis *et al.*, 2017).

4i.1.3 Hydroxyethyl starch

Hydroxyethyl starch (HES) is an umbrella term for all hydroxyethyl starches, which are subclassified based on their molecular structure (see Fig. 4i.1 for an example). HES products are manufactured through modification of amylopectin from maize or potato. Amylopectin is a polysaccharide consisting of long stretches of linked glucose units that branch at the C6 position of the glucose ring, every 20–25 glucose units (Green *et al.*, 1975). Natural polysaccharide solutions administered intravenously are rapidly degraded by amylases, thus are poor for sustained volume expansion. The substitution of hydroxyethyl groups ($-CH_2CH_2OH$) along the starch backbone modifies the rate of degradation by serum amylases, allowing for sustained volume expansion (DiBartola, 2012). HES molecules are broken down to eventually undergo primary renal

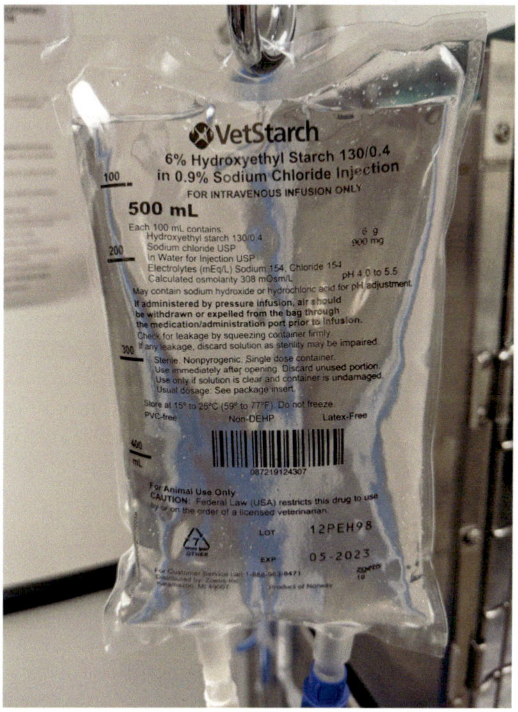

Fig. 4i.1. An image of VetStarch, a representative hydroxyethyl starch.

elimination; other routes of elimination include extravasation, interstitial storage sites, and biliary excretion (Wong and Koenig, 2017).

Certain properties of hydroxyethyl starches affect the pharmacokinetics/pharmacodynamics and have been awarded specific nomenclature (Fig. 4i.2), discussed below.

Mean molecular weight

Most HES products will contain a polydispersion of molecular sizes ranging from 10 kDa to >1000 kDa (Glover *et al.*, 2014). The molecular weight (MW) of a solution may be described as **number-averaged** MW (total weight of polymer divided by number of molecules) or **weight-averaged** MW, which is calculated through analysis of the fraction of total mass each molecular size contributes. It is the latter that will often be displayed on the HES packaging. Newer-generation HES solutions have smaller molecular weight features, but available products may range from 70 kDa to 670 kDa (Glover *et al.*, 2014). Circulating larger molecules may increase the side-effect profile and act as a reservoir to feed the pool of oncotically active molecules (Westphal *et al.*, 2009). Smaller molecules at the lower limit of renal threshold (45–60 kDa) are rapidly excreted in patients with normal renal function (Adamik *et al.*, 2015).

Degree of substitution, molar substitution

The frequency of hydroxyethyl substitution along the glucose ring (i.e., sites C_2, C_3, C_6) is directly proportional to solubility and inversely proportional to rate of degradation. **Degree of substitution** represents this frequency and is calculated as the number of anhydrous glucose units containing substitutions divided by the total number of anhydrous glucose units. A similar assessment known as the **molar substitution** accounts for the average number of hydroxyethyl substitutions per ten anhydroglucose units. This value is displayed as a decimal and determines prefix nomenclature (e.g., Hetastarch-0.7, Hexastarch-0.6, etc.). Additionally, a higher degree of substitution is correlated to a slower rate of degradation, as more obstacles are created for α-amylase in accessing intermolecular bonds (Westphal *et al.*, 2009; Glover *et al.*, 2014).

Pattern of substitution – C_2/C_6 ratio

Hydroxyethyl groups are substituted predominantly at the C_2 and C_6 positions along the glucose ring (Fig. 4i.3). Glucose molecules may have zero to three hydroxyethyl groups (DiBartola, 2012). Hydroxyethyl groups at the C_2 residue inhibit the action of α-amylase to the linking bonds more readily than those at the C_6 position, thus solutions with high C_2/C_6 ratios exhibit a slower rate of degradation. Comparative studies of different HES products that differ only in their C_2/C_6 ratio show that the ratio alone has significant impact on the area under plasma concentration curves (Westphal *et al.*, 2009).

Concentration

The concentration of a solution is determined from mass per unit volume (g/l) of starch molecules. Mass per unit may be influenced by both number of molecules and size of molecules. With that being said, it is the *number* of molecules that influences a solution's colloid osmotic pressure (COP) and determines the initial volume expanding effect. This is clinically relevant, as small molecules are extravasated or secreted within hours of administration, leading to short durations of volume expansion—shorter than what is often reported in manufacturers'

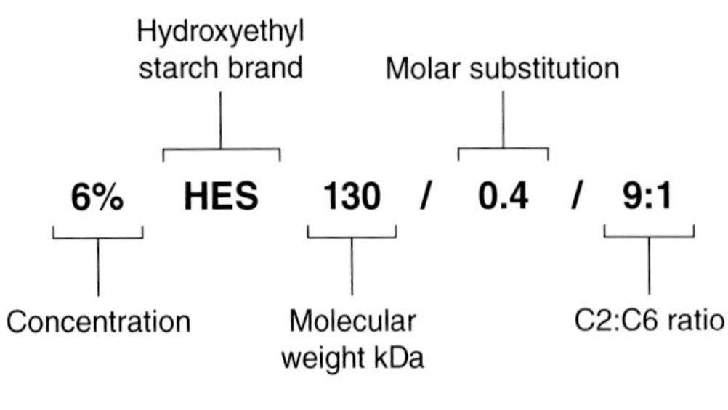

Fig. 4i.2. Hydroxyethyl starch nomenclature. (© The Ohio State University.)

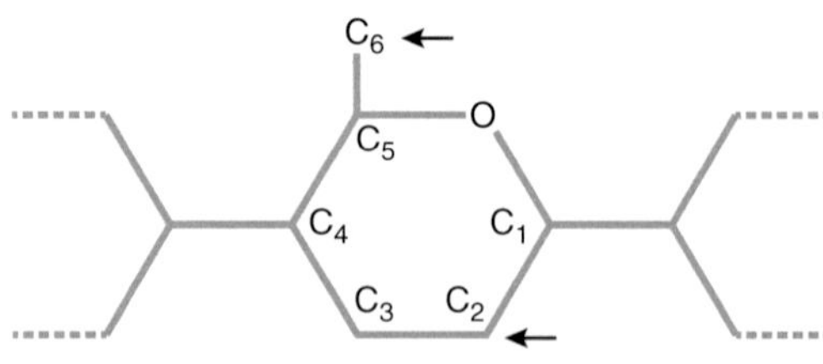

Fig. 4i.3. Substitutions of hydroxyethyl groups ($-CH_2CH_2OH$) for hydroxyl groups (-OH) take place preferentially at the C_2 and C_6 positions of the glucose ring (arrows). (© The Ohio State University.)

data sheets (DiBartola, 2012). Volume expansion or improvements in COP may be even further blunted in states of hypoalbuminemia and capillary leak syndromes (Veneman *et al.*, 2004; Borrelli *et al.*, 2020). Commercial solutions are available as 3%, 6%, and 10% solutions.

4i.2 Pharmacokinetics and Pharmacodynamics

Degradation of HES molecules and their *in vivo* half-life are determined by serum amylase activity and features of their molecular structure (i.e., degree and pattern of substitution) (Cazzolli and Prittie, 2015). Large HES molecules >60 kDa require enzymatic degradation by hydrolytic α-amylase or via the reticuloendothelial system; it has been published that dogs have higher levels of α-amylase as compared with humans (Glover *et al.*, 2014). Up to 70% of smaller molecules (≤55–60 kDa) undergo renal elimination, while the remainder of molecules may enter intracellular or interstitial spaces (Glover *et al.*, 2014). Lysosomal enzymes lack amylases, however, and possess less efficient α-glucosidases, which slowly degrade intracellular starch deposits into glucose (Adamik *et al.*, 2015; Cazzolli and Prittie, 2015).

In the presence of an intact endothelial glycocalyx (EG) and endothelial surface layer (ESL), HES solutions are theoretically limited to the intravascular space. This phenomenon is explained by the modification of the Starling hypothesis. The original **Starling hypothesis** described net transvascular fluid fluxes as a balance between the hydrostatic and oncotic pressures that exist between the intravascular and interstitial spaces. The modified version of this concept incorporates the dramatic role played by the ESL and the subglyceal space it creates (see Chapter 2 for additional information). The low COP of the subglyceal space counters that of the intravascular lumen, generating a large gradient that minimizes fluid extravasation under steady-state conditions (Gaudette *et al.*, 2020). Albumin concentrated within superficial layers of the ESL appears necessary to the integrity of the endothelial surface layer. Furthermore, albumin's role in preventing vascular leak independently of its COP is known as the "COP paradox" (Adamik *et al.*, 2015).

Several studies have evaluated the effects of albumin and HES on transvascular fluid flux in the presence of a healthy and degraded ESL (Smiley and Garvey, 1994; Jacob *et al.*, 2006, 2007). In the presence of a normal ESL, albumin and HES alike attenuate transcapillary leak. Interestingly, albumin outperformed HES in conditions of ascending hydrostatic pressures or increased permeability despite HES generating a higher COP as compared with albumin. Both natural and synthetic colloids equilibrate with the interstitial space; however, the kinetic transport of albumin across an intact vascular wall is approximately 20% that of HES. This suggests an overall reduced vascular permeability to albumin compared with HES despite its smaller molecular weight. This phenomenon is likely referable to the charged nature of albumin versus the neutral nature of HES, and the barrier provided by the negatively charged ESL. In further support of this, states of severely damaged ESL (i.e., post-ischemia plus enzymatic destruction) result in complete inability for albumin and HES to prevent capillary leak (Jacob *et al.*, 2006, 2007). These findings are translational, as ischemia and ESL/endothelial cell damage may occur in a number of clinical situations, including surgery, sepsis, hemorrhagic shock, hypervolemia, and hyperglycemia (Aldecoa *et al.*, 2020).

4i.3 Adverse Risk Profile of Semi-synthetic Colloids

4i.3.1 Coagulopathy

Large-volume intravenous fluid therapy of any type can impair coagulation through dilution of hemostatic proteins and platelets. This effect is notable when isotonic crystalloids achieve dilutions of whole blood approximating 33% and hypertonic saline achieves dilutions of whole blood approximating 8% (Chan *et al.*, 2020). The coagulopathy associated with synthetic colloid use is likely multifactorial, including reduced platelet function (i.e., colloid-osmotic shrinking of platelets), reduced platelet adhesion and aggregation (i.e. altered reduced expression of platelet receptor GPIIbIIIa), dilution of coagulation factors, reduced FVIIIa/vWF interactions, diminished vWF-mediated rolling, reduced clot strength, and enhanced fibrinolysis (DiBartola, 2012; Adamik *et al.*, 2015). In addition, HES products with high MS or C_2/C_6 ratios are expected to have longer half-lives, thus accumulating more readily, causing more profound effects on coagulation disturbances. Molecular weight is thought to have less impact on coagulation impairment (Adamik *et al.*, 2015). Coagulopathy associated with synthetic colloid use is known to be dose-dependent, leading to manufacturers' recommended maximal daily dosing (see Table 4i.1) (Cazzolli and Prittie, 2015). Furthermore, more dramatic coagulation disturbances are observed with the combination of HES and hypertonic saline (Chan *et al.*, 2020). A meta-analysis in 2018 evaluated 69 studies to find moderate-certainty evidence that starches slightly increased the need for blood transfusion (Lewis *et al.*, 2018). Gelatin and dextran solution have demonstrated similar coagulation derangements (Cazzolli and Prittie, 2015).

4i.3.2 Kidney injury

Several human randomized control trials (RCTs) have demonstrated that HES use increases the risk of AKI and the need for renal replacement therapy (RRT) and increases mortality, particularly in those with sepsis (Glover *et al.*, 2014; Unal and Reinhart, 2019). Meta-analysis data reported in 2018 showed an increased relative risk for RRT with the use of HES, but conclusions could not be drawn with regard to dextrans or gelatins (Lewis *et al.*, 2018). As such, in human patients the use of synthetic colloids is considered contraindicated in almost all clinical circumstances (Rhodes *et al.*, 2017). The exact mechanism of renal injury remains unclear, but is likely multifactorial (Fig. 4i.4). One contributing factor is related to reabsorption of HES macromolecules into proximal renal tubular cells leading to **osmotic nephrosis** (ON). The term ON describes a histomorphological pattern (i.e., intracytoplasmic vacuolization, proximal tubular swelling) that is considered non-specific and may be seen with other hyperosmolar intravenous agents (e.g., intravenous immunoglobulin, mannitol, iodine contrast media) (Glover *et al.*, 2014; Schmid *et al.*, 2019). Several human and canine studies have documented ON-like lesions secondary to HES use, but evidence of the clinical relevance of these findings in veterinary medicine has been sparse. One study found that although lesions of ON could be found in dogs who received starches and those who did not, cumulative HES dose (6% HES 670/0.75) was a significant predictor of tubular vacuolization (Schmid *et al.*, 2019). An additional theory is that of **hyperoncotic AKI,** in which an increased COP antagonizes hydrostatic pressure and decreases glomerular filtration rate. This effect would be most prominent with higher-concentration HES

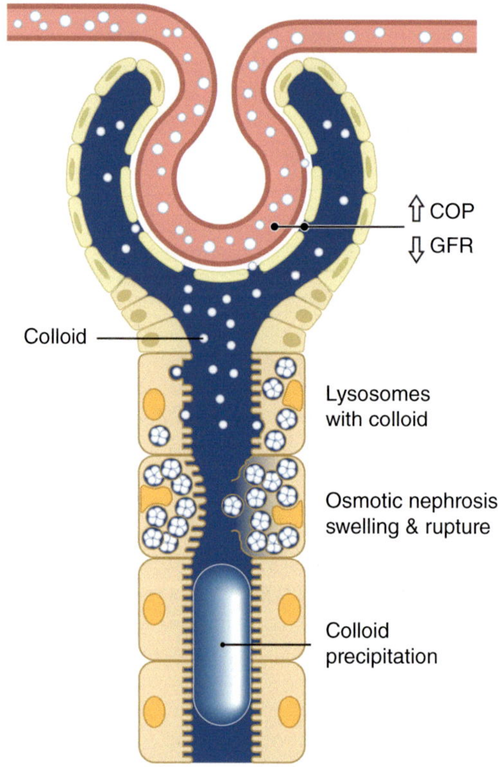

Fig. 4i.4. Schematic diagram highlighting the potential causes of kidney injury associated with administration of synthetic colloids. Increased oncotic pressure can result in decreased GFR. Lysosome accumulation in tubular epithelial cells can lead to crowding and dysfunction, ultimately leading to rupture from swelling secondary to osmotic nephrosis. Finally, colloid molecules can accumulate and obstruct the tubular lumen. (© The Ohio State University.)

solutions (i.e., 10% HES), as molecular weight and molar substitution have little effect on COP. This theory has been contested by meta-analysis data that demonstrated it is likely to be the specific properties of the colloid molecule (HES versus albumin), rather than the concentration, that determine deleterious renal effects (Wiedermann *et al.*, 2010).

The veterinary literature is inconclusive with regard to HES use and associated risk of AKI in cats (Sigrist *et al.*, 2017; Yozova *et al.*, 2017) and dogs (Zersen *et al.*, 2019). Studies are difficult to compare, due to differences in HES generation use, cumulative dose, variable or absent illness severity scoring, definitions of AKI, and discrepancies in how species metabolize various colloid solutions. It is currently recommended in the human literature to use balanced crystalloids as first line therapy for resuscitation and maintenance in any patient at risk or with established AKI, with avoidance of synthetic colloids (Perner *et al.*, 2017; Ostermann *et al.*, 2019).

4i.3.3 Sepsis and capillary leak syndromes

In systemic inflammatory disease states, defects in components of the microcirculation may result in changes in vascular permeability. As previously mentioned, the "leakiness" of the ESL may be altered by certain inflammatory conditions such as surgery, trauma, or sepsis (Finfer, 2013). Inflammatory mediators may result in endothelial cell contraction and altered endothelial cell junctions (Glover *et al.*, 2014). Additionally, inflammatory mediator-induced enzymatic destruction or hypervolemia results in damage to the endothelial glycocalyx scaffold and abnormal vascular permeability (Salmon and Satchell, 2012; Aldecoa *et al.*, 2020). Theories of reinforcement of the EG scaffold with hydroxyethyl starches have been explored since the 1980s (Jacob *et al.*, 2006; Glover *et al.*, 2014). HES may function as a rudimentary contributor to the EG scaffold; however, in post-ischemic states or following EG enzymatic destruction, this effect is significantly blunted, reinforcing the concept that HES attenuation of capillary leak relies on an intact ESL (Jacob *et al.*, 2006). As such, predictable pharmacokinetics of synthetic colloids are not reliable in inflammatory states of increased vascular permeability. Liberal use of synthetic colloids in such circumstances may result in increased extravasation of synthetic colloid solutions, perpetuation of interstitial edema, worsening of oxygen delivery to tissues, and organ dysfunction (Zazzeron *et al.*, 2016).

4i.4 Indications and Contraindications

Hydroxyethyl starches continue to be the most utilized and available colloid in the USA. Regarding HES use in critically ill human populations, the contraindications list far exceeds the indications list (Table 4i.2). This has to do with extensive research in critically ill populations showing increased risk of AKI, RRT, and mortality as previously indicated (Unal and Reinhart, 2019). Although it can be debated if the human literature can be directly extrapolated to veterinary patients, due to differences in metabolism (i.e., increased canine α-amylase activity), strong evidence of efficacy is lacking. Attention should be given to patient selection and cumulative dose administration (Wong and Koenig, 2017). Further explanations of indications, cautions, and contraindications are provided below.

4i.4.1 Acute volume expansion

While avoiding patients affected by conditions highlighted in Table 4i.2, appropriate candidates who may benefit from acute volume expansion with hydroxyethyl starches include peri-operative patients, emergency patients in acute hypovolemic shock secondary to marked GI losses (e.g., acute severe vomiting), obstructive shock (e.g., GDV) or reduced effective circulating volume (e.g., anaphylaxis) (Glover *et al.*, 2014). See Chapter 6i for additional information regarding use of synthetic colloids in acute volume expansion.

4i.4.2 Hypoalbuminemia

It has been historically accepted that synthetic colloids are effective in supporting oncotic pressure in order to reduce extravasation of crystalloid therapy and reduce peripheral edema. Although one study of hypoalbuminemic dogs has documented subjective improvement in edema with the use of HES, resolution of edema was not correlated to COP, dose of HES or survival (Smiley and Garvey, 1994). Critical review of the HES literature is more controversial than confident regarding any sustained impact on COP or positive outcome measure in patients that suffer from low baseline COP (Moore and Garvey, 1996; Borrelli *et al.*, 2020).

Given that hypoalbuminemia is often associated with chronic disease or critical illness, one must consider the etiology of the hypoalbuminemia in order to make decisions about appropriate patient

Table 4i.2. List of indications and contraindications for hydroxyethyl starch.

Indications	Contraindications
Acute volume expansion	Renal impairment/Risk for AKI
+/– Hypoalbuminemia	Coagulopathy
	Sepsis/Critical illness
	Burn patients
	Pulmonary edema
	Cardiac insufficiency
	Intracranial hypertension
	Severe liver disease
	Hypervolemia

selection for HES use. More recent recommendations regarding treatment of hypoalbuminemia in veterinary medicine stray away from correcting a value; rather, they emphasize addressing the underlying disease (loss versus lack of production versus consumption), practicing judicious crystalloid use, and utilizing early enteral nutrition (Conner, 2017). In resource-limited settings in which a hypoalbuminemic patient is experiencing signs of hypovolemic shock (i.e., tachycardia, weak pulse quality, dull mentation), acute resuscitation with colloid therapy (3–5 ml/kg IV bolus over 20–30 min) may be appropriate. Given the concerns for cumulative effects on coagulation, tissue storage, and kidney injury, continuous-rate infusions of synthetic colloids should be avoided. Instead, application of enteral nutrition and judicious crystalloid use should be considered as standard of care in hemodynamically stable hypoalbuminemic patients. Patients with complex disease or protracted critical illness may benefit from albumin-containing products, which has been reviewed elsewhere (Mazzaferro and Edwards, 2020). See also Chapter 4ii for additional information on use of natural colloids.

4i.5 Summary

Considering the complex relationships between COP, capillary leak and colloid extravasation, patient selection becomes the most crucial decision when establishing fluid therapy plans. The goal to increase effective circulating volume may quickly become futile in the face of a compromised ESL as a result of enhanced colloid extravasation, interstitial edema, and suppression of albumin synthesis (Adamik *et al.*, 2015). With concerns for suboptimal efficacy and adverse events, synthetic colloid use is often restricted to situations of acute volume expansion in states of low effective circulating volume in non-coagulopathic and non-renal impaired states. In human patients with severe inflammatory disease states and sepsis, crystalloids are the preferred solution for resuscitation, as semi-synthetic colloids have largely fallen out of favor due to increased risk of morbidity and mortality. Strong evidence-based recommendations are less available in veterinary medicine without extrapolation from human data. As such, at the author's institution, judicious synthetic colloid therapy may be considered for stabilization during diagnostic acquisition and interventional planning. However, prolonged infusions are avoided and preference is afforded to lower-risk management plans, including judicious crystalloids, enteral nutrition, and natural colloids. Such strategies are especially relevant to the critically ill patient, as observations of *in vitro* and *in vivo* studies have demonstrated that albumin and fresh frozen plasma are superior to crystalloids and artificial colloids in their ability to protect and restore the ESL (Aldecoa *et al.*, 2020).

References

Adamik, K.N., Yozova, I.D. and Regenscheit, N. (2015) Controversies in the use of hydroxyethyl starch solutions in small animal emergency and critical care. *Journal of Veterinary Emergency and Critical Care* 25, 20–47.

Aldecoa, C., Llau, J.V., Nuvials, X. *et al.* (2020) Role of albumin in the preservation of endothelial glycocalyx integrity and the microcirculation: a review. *Annals of Intensive Care* 10, 85.

Borrelli, A., Maurella, C., Lippi, I. *et al.* (2020) Evaluation of the effects of hydroxyethyl starch (130/0.4) administration as a constant rate infusion on plasma colloid osmotic pressure in hypoabluminemic dogs. *Journal of Veterinary Emergency and Critical Care* 30, 550–557.

Brown, R.M. and Semler, M.W. (2019) Fluid management in sepsis. *Journal of Intensive Care Medicine* 34, 364–373.

Casey, J.D., Brown, R.M. and Semler, M.W. (2018) Resuscitation fluids. *Current Opinions in Critical Care* 24, 512–518.

Cazzolli, D. and Prittie, J. (2015) The crystalloid–colloid debate: consequences of resuscitation fluid selection in veterinary critical care. *Journal of Veterinary Emergency and Critical Care* 25, 6–19.

Chan, A., Hughes, D., Tennent-brown, B.S. *et al.* (2020) In vitro effects of lactated Ringer's solution, hypertonic saline, hydroxyethyl starch, hypertonic saline/hydroxyethyl starch, and mannitol on thromboelastographic variables of canine whole blood. *Journal of Veterinary Emergency and Critical Care* 30, 255–263.

Conner, B.J. (2017) Treating hypoalbuminemia. *Veterinary Clinics of North America Small Animal Practice* 47, 451–459.

DiBartola, S.P. (2012) *Fluid, Electrolyte, and Acid-Base Disorders in Small Animal Practice*, 4th edn. Saunders/Elsevier, St Louis, Missouri.

Drobatz, K.J., Hopper, K., Rozanski, E.A. and Silverstein, D.C. (2019) *Textbook of Small Animal Emergency Medicine*, 2nd edn. Elsevier, St Louis, Missouri.

Finfer, S. (2013) Reappraising the role of albumin for resuscitation. *Current Opinions in Critical Care* 19(4), 315–320.

Gaudette, S., Hughes, D. and Boller, M. (2020) The endothelial glycocalyx: structure and function in health and critical illness. *Journal of Veterinary Emergency and Critical Care* 30, 117–134.

Glover, P.A., Rudloff, E. and Kirby, R. (2014) Hydroxyethyl starch: a review of pharmacokinetics, pharmacodynamics, current products, and potential clinical risks, benefits, and use. *Journal of Veterinary Emergency and Critical Care* 24, 642–661.

Green, M.M., Blankenhorn, G. and Hart, H. (1975) Textbook Errors, 123 – Which starch fraction is water-soluble, amylose or amylopectin? *Journal of Chemical Education* 52, 729–730.

Grimm, K.A., Lamont, L.A., Tranquilli, W.J. *et al.* (eds) (2015) *Veterinary Anesthesia and Analgesia*, 5th edn. John Wiley & Sons Inc., Ames, Iowa.

Jacob, M., Bruegger, D., Rehm, M. *et al.* (2006) Contrasting effects of colloid and crystalloid resuscitation fluids on cardiac vascular permeability. *Anesthesiology* 104, 1223–1231.

Jacob, M., Bruegger, D., Rehm, M. *et al.* (2007) The endothelial glycocalyx affords compatibility of Starling's principle and high cardiac interstitial albumin levels. *Cardiovascular Research* 73, 575–586.

Joannidis, M., Druml, W., Forni, L.G. *et al.* (2017) Prevention of acute kidney injury and protection of renal function in the intensive care unit: update 2017. Expert opinion of the Working Group on Prevention, AKI section, European Society of Intensive Care Medicine. *Intensive Care Medicine* 43, 730–749.

Lewis, S.R., Pritchard, M.W., Evans, D.J. *et al.* (2018) Colloids versus crystalloids for fluid resuscitation in critically ill people. *Cochrane Database of Systematic Reviews* 8, CD000567.

Mazzaferro, E.M. and Edwards, T. (2020) Update on albumin therapy in critical illness. *Veterinary Clinics of North America Small Animal Practice* 50, 1289–1305.

Moore, L.E. and Garvey, M.S. (1996) The effect of hetastarch on serum colloid oncotic pressure in hypoalbuminemic dogs. *Journal of Veterinary Internal Medicine* 10, 300–303.

Ostermann, M., Liu, K. and Kashani, K. (2019) Fluid management in acute kidney injury. *Chest* 156, 594–603.

Perner, A., Prowle, J., Joannidis, M. *et al.* (2017) Fluid management in acute kidney injury. *Intensive Care Medicine* 44, 807–815.

Rhodes, A., Evans, L.E. and Alhazzani, W. (2017) Surviving Sepsis Campaign: International Guidelines for Management of Sepsis and Septic Shock: 2016. *Intensive Care Medicine* 43, 304–377.

Rozga, J., Piatek, T. and Malkowski, P. (2013) Human albumin: old, new, and emerging applications. *Annals of Transplantation* 18, 205–217.

Salmon, A.H. and Satchell, S.C. (2012) Endothelial glycocalyx dysfunction in disease: albuminuria and increased microvascular permeability. *Journal of Patholology* 226, 562–574.

Schmid, S.M., Cianciolo, R.E., Drobatz, K.J. *et al.* (2019) Postmortem evaluation of renal tubular vacuolization in critically ill dogs. *Journal of Veterinary Emergency and Critical Care* 29, 279–287.

Schott, U., Kander, T. and Bentzer, P. (2018) Effects of Dextran-70 and albumin on coagulation in experimental hemorrhage in the guinea pig. *Shock* 50, 366–372.

Sigrist, N.E., Kalin, N. and Dreyfus, A. (2017) Effects of hydroxyethyl starch 130/0.4 on serum creatinine concentration and development of acute kidney injury in nonazotemic cats. *Journal of Veterinary Internal Medicine* 31, 1749–1756.

Smiley, L.E. and Garvey, M.S. (1994) The use of hetastarch as adjunct therapy in 26 dogs with hypoalbuminemia: a phase two clinical trial. *Journal of Veterinary Internal Medicine* 8, 195–202.

Unal, M.N. and Reinhart, K. (2019) Understanding the harms of HES: a review of the evidence to date. *Turkish Journal of Anaesthesiology and Reanimation* 47, 81–91.

Veneman, T.F., Oude Nijhuis, J. and Woittiez, A.J. (2004) Human albumin and starch administration in critically ill patients: a prospective randomized clinical trial. *Wiener Klinische Wochenschrift* 116, 305–309.

Westphal, M., James, M.F., Kozek-Langenecker, S. *et al.* (2009) Hydroxyethyl starches: different products – different effects. *Anesthesiology* 111, 187–202.

Wiedermann, C.J., Dunzendorfer, S., Gaioni, L.U. *et al.* (2010) Hypertonic colloids and acute kidney injury: a meta-analysis of randomized trials. *Critical Care* 14(5), R191.

Wong, C. and Koenig, A. (2017) The colloid controversy: are colloids bad and what are the options? *Veterinary Clinics of North America Small Animal Practice* 47, 411–421.

Yozova, I.D., Howard, J. and Adamik, K.N. (2017) Effect of tetrastarch (hydroxyethyl starch 130/0.4) on plasma creatinine concentration in cats: a retrospective analysis (2010–2015). *Journal of Feline Medicine and Surgery* 19, 1073–1079.

Zazzeron, L., Gattiononi, L. and Caironi, P. (2016) Role of albumin, starches and gelatins versus crystalloids in volume resuscitation of critically ill patients. *Current Opinions in Critical Care* 22, 428–436.

Zersen, K.M., Mama, K. and Mathis, J.C. (2019) Retrospective evaluation of paired plasma creatinine and chloride concentrations following hetastarch administration in anesthetized dogs (2002–2015): 244 cases. *Journal of Veterinary Emergency and Critical Care* 29, 309–313.

4ii Natural Colloids

JULIEN GUILLAUMIN

Colorado State University, Fort Collins, Colorado, USA

Fluid administration is a very important part of medicine and understanding the various types of fluid is the cornerstone of the clinician's ability to choose the appropriate fluid type for a patient. Although isotonic crystalloids are generally safe, inexpensive, and ubiquitous in clinical practice, they may not be appropriate for all patients. In the previous section of this chapter (Chapter 4i) the stage was set regarding potential applications for colloid administration, and specifics regarding synthetic colloids. This section (Chapter 4ii) will be focused on the different types and use of natural colloids, which are protein particles (e.g., albumin) suspended in a liquid plasma phase. As these larger molecules are more likely to remain in the vascular compartment, they confer **colloid osmotic pressure** (COP), also known as oncotic pressure (Chan, 2008), and can thereby contribute to circulating volume. In addition, provision of natural colloids can also support some of the other vital functions that albumin serves.

4ii.1 Types of Plasma Products Available

Fresh whole blood (FWB) is the root plasma-containing fluid from which the other products are derived. While FWB could be used as a natural colloid, this is not typically recommended unless there is need for concurrent red blood cell administration (such as the hemorrhaging patient), or other plasma products are not available. The most commonly used plasma product from FWB is **fresh frozen plasma** (FFP). A unit of FFP comes from a fresh whole blood donation, when the red blood cell component has been separated (Fig. 4ii.1). It is then frozen within 6–8 h of collection and stored for less than 1-2 years at below −22°F (−30°C) in order to be considered FFP. Frozen plasma (FP) is FFP that has been stored for more than 1–2 years or is frozen more than 6–8 h after collection. Frozen plasma is thought to be depleted of co-factors V and VIII, although this notion from human medicine has been challenged in veterinary medicine (Urban *et al.*, 2013). Essentially, while there may be a decrease in the activity of these factors, there is still sufficient quantity to support normal coagulation. Both products can be used for the provision of albumin and coagulation factors. The maximum storage length for FFP/FP is 5 years (Davidow, 2013).

Fresh frozen plasma can be further divided in **cryoprecipitate** (cryo) and **cryoprecipitate-poor** (cryo-poor) plasma (CPP), because different factors have different freezing points. Cryoprecipitate is made by partially thawing FFP at 39°F (4°C) for 24 h and removing the supernatant. This leaves the semi-solid cryoprecipitate, containing factor VIII, fibrinogen, and **von Willebrand factor** (vWf). Cryoprecipitate is indicated for bleeding associated with vWf deficiency or hemophilia A, as well as patients with hypofibrinogenemia (e.g., exsanguination) (Davidow, 2013). The supernatant is CPP, also known as **cryosupernatant** or **cryo-depleted plasma.** CPP is indicated for use in vitamin K antagonist rodenticide toxicities and hypoalbuminemia (Davidow, 2013). Albumin can also be separated and concentrated from FFP. Albumin solutions will be covered later in the chapter. The components of various plasma products are listed in Tables 4ii.1 and 4ii.2.

4ii.2 Indications to Use Natural Colloids as a Fluid

4ii.2.1 Provision of clotting factors and volume expansion

The main indications for FFP transfusion are treatment of coagulopathies such as anticoagulant rodenticide intoxication, Hemophilia A or B: the trigger is evidence of clinical bleeding (e.g., dropping hematocrit, active bleeding) with severe increase of the

DOI: 10.1079/9781789243406.0042

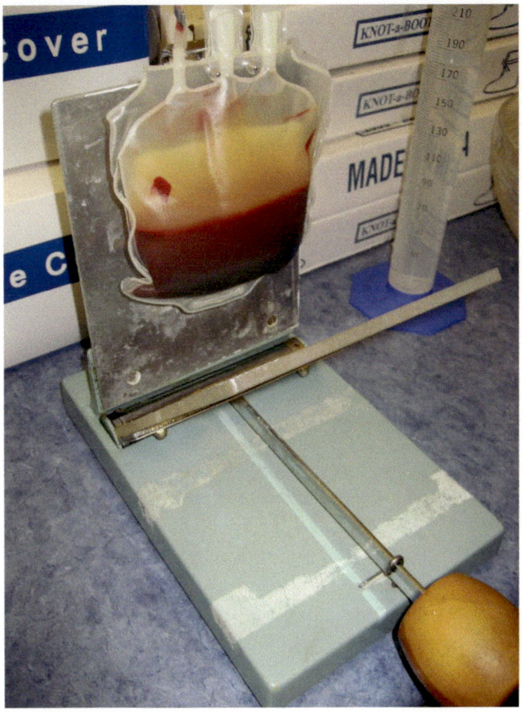

Fig. 4ii.1. After fresh whole blood (FWB) collection, the FWB bag is placed in a blood product-specific centrifuge to separate the red blood cells component from the liquid/plasma phase component. The plasma can be moved to a transfer bag using pressure generated by a cell separator (shown).

clotting times, usually activated partial thromboplastin time (or activated clotting time) and prothrombin time (Fig. 4ii.2). The volume needed for replacement of clotting factors for patients with clinical bleeding due to a coagulopathy is usually FFP at 10–20 ml/kg, or FWB at 20–40 ml/kg. The dose of cryoprecipitate is usually 1 unit (approximately 70–100 mL per 10 kg). The dose for CPP is 10–20 mL/kg depending on the indication (i.e. coagulopathy vs albumin replacement). See Clinical Case 4ii.1 for an example of plasma used for this purpose. It is considered an inappropriate use of FFP to treat increased clotting times without evidence of clinical bleeding (including for a minor procedure), or for α-macroglobulins replacement in pancreatitis, or anti-thrombin replacement in disseminated intravascular coagulation (Rozanski *et al.*, 2001; Davidow, 2013).

Plasma products like FFP can also be used in acute volume expansion, particularly in hypoproteinemic patients. Another consideration is volume replacement fluid in exsanguinating patients potentially needing massive transfusion. In these circumstances FFP transfusion is provided at a recommended ratio of 1:1 with packed red blood cells (Sihler and Napolitano, 2009). In that case, the volume transfused may reach a total of approximately 20–40 ml/kg and potentially more.

4ii.2.2 Albumin supplementation

For the purpose of ongoing fluid administration, the main indication to use a plasma product is to provide species-specific albumin replacement and oncotic support. Albumin is one of the most important proteins in the body. Its physiologic functions are numerous, including transport proteins for many elements (e.g., hormones, drugs), free-radical scavenging, maintenance of the oncotic pressure (albumin is responsible for 70–80% of normal oncotic pressure), anti-apoptotic effects, anticoagulant and anti-thrombotic, acid–base buffering, and anti-inflammatory properties (Craft and Powell, 2012; Rozga *et al.*, 2013).

Albumin is a small molecule (66 kDa), synthetized by the liver. Hepatic onco-receptors regulate its synthesis. The usual quoted volume of distribution is 30% intravascular and 70% extravascular, but the transcapillary rate is very slow, as it can take several days for albumin to move across the endothelial membrane. After albumin infusion to healthy patients, 90% is still intravascular after 2 h, and 25% after 2 days. However, that transcapillary flux can be increased up to 13 times in critical illness (e.g., infection, shock, burns). Moreover, albumin's half-life (8.2 days in dogs) is inversely dependent on its concentration, with hypoalbuminemia increasing its half-life (Boldt, 2010).

It is well documented that hypoalbuminemia carries a worse prognosis in critically ill humans. Each 1.0 g/dl decrease in albumin increases the odds of mortality by 137% and morbidity by 89% (Vincent, 2009). This is also documented in veterinary medicine (Roux *et al.*, 2013). Although hypoalbuminemia is a risk factor for death and worsening illness, the link between albumin replacement and improved outcome continues to be debated. In humans, there is evidence that albumin replacement does not improve mortality for perioperative patients, in heterogenous ICU population, or in trauma patients (Boldt, 2010; Roberts *et al.*, 2011; SAFE Study Investigators, 2011). Albumin transfusion is contra-indicated in traumatic brain injury patients

Table 4ii.1. Types of blood products, and their components, available in veterinary medicine (based on data from Culler *et al.*, 2017).

Blood product	Contents	Applications
Fresh whole blood	Red blood cells, clotting factors, albumin, immunoglobulins, plasma	Hemorrhage Severe anemia Coagulopathy
Fresh frozen plasma (FFP)	Clotting factors, albumin, immunoglobulins, plasma	Coagulopathy Volume expansion Albumin replacement
Frozen plasma (>1 year or >6 h)	Clotting factors (except FV and FVIII)[a], immunoglobulins, albumin plasma	Coagulopathy (except Hemophilia A)[a] Volume expansion Albumin replacement
Cryoprecipitate	Factor I (fibrinogen), Factor VIII, Factor IX, von Willebrand factor	Coagulopathy, especially Hemophilia A and vWf deficiency Source of fibrinogen in case of massive transfusion
Cryo-poor plasma	Factors other than VIII, XIII, I, and vWf. Contains low levels of Factor IX, with a 68% activity. Albumin (3.2 g/dl)	May still be suitable for anti-vitamin K factor deficiency Should not be used for Hemophilia A, vWf deficiency, and probably Hemophilia B Source of albumin more important compared with FFP or cryoprecipitate
Concentrated albumin (5–25%)	Albumin	Albumin replacement in selected situations

[a] This notion has been challenged in veterinary medicine by Urban *et al.* (2013).

Table 4ii.2: Physiological characteristics and clinical effects of commonly used intravenous solutions. (Adapted from Ewalenko *et al.*, 1986; American Thoracic Society, 2004; Culler *et al.*, 2017)

	Albumin solution (4–5%)	Albumin solution (25%)	Fresh frozen plasma	0.9% NaCl
Molecular weight, average (kD)	69	69	FFP is 60% albumin	0
Osmolality (mOsm/l)	290	310	350	310
COP (mm Hg)	20–30	70–100	12.7	0
Plasmatic half-life (h)	16–24	16–24	Similar to albumin	0.3–0.5

(SAFE Study Investigators, 2011). Potential indications for albumin transfusion in humans are burns (Rozga *et al.*, 2013) and severe sepsis/septic shock (SAFE Study Investigators, 2011; Caironi *et al.*, 2014).

Veterinary sources of albumin are canine-specific albumin (CSA), or albumin contained in FFP (Craft and Powell, 2012). One veterinary blood bank sells a vial containing 5 g of lyophilized albumin and can be reconstituted as a 5% to 16% solution depending on the volume of diluent used (Animal Blood Resources International, available at: https://www.abrint.net/wp-content/uploads/2019/12/PACKAGE-INSERT-ALB.pdf, accessed 2 December 2020). The dose suggested on the package insert is 0.45–0.8 g/kg over 4–8 h. The albumin content of FFP is relatively low, around 2.9 g/dl (corresponding to 2.9% albumin). Therefore, a target of supplementing 0.8 g/kg will require FFP at 27 ml/kg, which can easily be delivered over a few hours or as a constant rate infusion. Using cryo-poor plasma will reduce the total volume, as it contains a higher albumin content than FFP (Culler *et al.*, 2019). The use of cryo-poor plasma as an albumin replacement fluid, given as a constant rate infusion (CRI), has been published in veterinary medicine (Ropski *et al.*, 2017; Culler *et al.*, 2019). Many veterinary references use a specific formula to calculate the dose of albumin to be given. That dose in grams is based on the formula 10 × desired delta albumin × weight (kg) × 0.3, but the origin of that formula points to albumin replacement using total parenteral nutrition in the 1980s (Brown *et al.*, 1987). Based on this calculation, it would take albumin at 1.5 g/kg (amounting to plasma at 50 ml/kg) to achieve an increase of 0.5 g/dl. However, most studies in people investigating albumin use for critically ill patients use a fixed

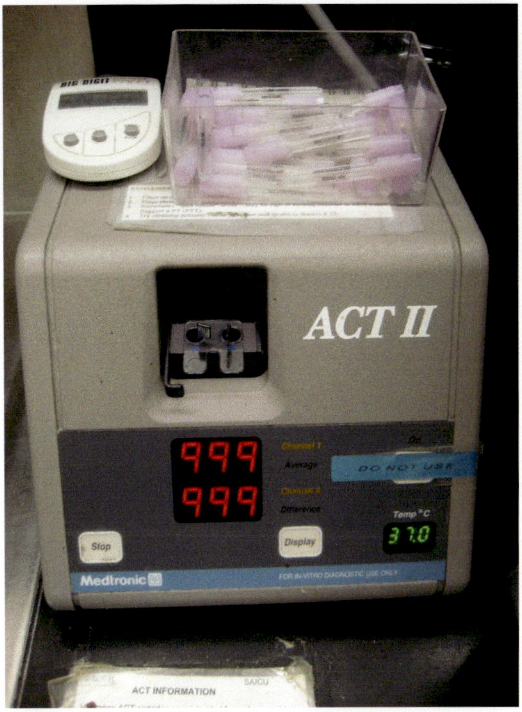

Fig. 4ii.2. Severe coagulopathy, shown here by a severe increase of activated clotting time (ACT), associated with clinical evidence of bleeding, is one of the main indications for use of plasma products in small animals.

dose of albumin, ranging from 0.2 to 1 g/kg/day (SAFE Study Investigators, 2011; Caironi *et al.*, 2014). With this target, the volume of natural colloid over a full period of 24 h then becomes more manageable. For example, Culler *et al.* (2019) showed that cryo-poor plasma at 1.8 ml/kg/h was associated with a rise of albumin from 1.5 g/dl to 2.1 g/dl in a retrospective study of ten hypoalbuminemic dogs. Clinical Case 4ii.2 demonstrates application of this concept.

4ii.2.3 Practicality of FFP infusions

Fresh frozen plasma can be administered to patients over 4 h in normovolemic patients, or faster if hypovolemia is present and resuscitation is needed. If plasma product is used as a constant rate infusion, it can be given as a rate of 1-2 ml/kg/h (Ropski *et al.*, 2017). If this method of delivery is chosen, only 4–6 h of plasma should be set up on the fluid pump or syringe pump at a time. The volume needed should be aseptically removed or split from the storage bag, with the unused portion kept in the refrigerator until needed. The goal is to limit the potential for bacterial contamination.

Several methods have been described regarding thawing FFP. The most commonly used technique involves thawing in a warm-water bath at 98.6°F (37°C), which usually takes around 35–45 min. Although FFP has been thawed in a regular microwave oven using approximately 15 cycles of 10 seconds, and was shown to have similar activated partial thromboplastin times, the one-stage prothrombin times, concentrations of fibrinogen, factor-VIII coagulant activity, and vWf antigen levels compared with aliquots thawed in a warm-water bath, it is not the preferred methods of thawing (Hurst *et al.*, 1987). More recently, a study showed that a running-water bath had the shortest thaw time (15 min) compared with dry plasma thawer or warm-water bath, while maintaining clinically similar levels of hemostatic proteins (Torkildsen *et al.*, 2018). Commercially available microwave plasma defrosters allow for thawing in 3–5 min, while maintaining clinically relevant activities of clotting factors and fibrinogen concentration, although in this study no control group was used and some measurements of factor VIII activity fell below the reference interval (Turner *et al.*, 2018).

The use and hemostatic activity of liquid-phase (i.e., refrigerated) canine plasma has also been investigated. This product is used in humans with catastrophic hemorrhage needing massive transfusion, as it does not need to be thawed and is ready for rapid administration. It has been demonstrated that refrigerated storage results in significant decreases in the activity of all clotting factors, although no values were outside of the reference interval (Grochowsky *et al.*, 2014). Importantly, none of the bacterial cultures at days 7 and 14 yielded growth (Grochowsky *et al.*, 2014). The biggest potential limitation to the use of liquid phase plasma in veterinary cases is the potential to waste the product if not used within a 2-week period. Hospital caseload, acuity, and frequency of need would be the biggest determinants as to whether it is warranted to keep liquid phase plasma on hand.

4ii.2.4 Risks and adverse reactions to plasma transfusion

Transfusion reaction to plasma has been documented in a retrospective study of more than 300 canine plasma transfusions, in which the only side effects were fever, pruritis and anxiety. These were noted in less than 1% of cases (Snow *et al.*, 2010). This suggests that plasma transfusion, even with administration of multiple units, carries a very low risk of adverse events.

4ii.2.5 The use of human serum albumin (HSA)

The use of HSA (25%, or 250 mg/ml, or 0.25 g/ml) is an attractive solution to replenish albumin using lower volume, although the cost of HSA is still high. However, there is only 80% homology between CSA and HSA (Francis *et al.*, 2007). Therefore, transfusion of HSA to dogs will result in the production of anti-HSA antibodies, possibly leading to acute hypersensitivity reaction and death of HSA-transfused dogs re-exposed to HSA (Adamantos *et al.*, 2009). Moreover, approximately 8–10% of dogs have naturally occurring anti-HSA antibodies, so may develop an acute hypersensitivity reaction during their first HSA transfusion (Adamantos *et al.*, 2009). There are several reports on clinical use of HSA in dogs but concerns about immunization and acute (type I) and delayed (type III) hypersensitivity reactions limit its use. Further, using HSA multiple times in a patient is strictly contraindicated (Trow *et al.*, 2008; Adamantos *et al.*, 2009; Powell *et al.*, 2013). Also, it is documented that approximately 7% of critically ill dogs receiving HSA will have serious complications (Trow *et al.*, 2008; Viganó *et al.*, 2010). Therefore, clinicians must carefully weigh risk–benefits in individual patients before use.

4ii.3 Summary

Depending on the product selected, natural colloids can be used to provide acute support of circulating volume, correction of coagulopathy, and/or protein augmentation in hypoalbuminemic patients. Different options include FFP, FP, cryoprecipitate, CPP, CSA and HSA, each of which carries specific constituents and applications such that selection can be tailored to the patient's needs. Careful consideration of potential adverse effects, as well as cost and availability, should also impact the decision-making process.

Clinical Case 4ii.1

Molly is a female intact 2-year-old Australian shepherd dog who is presented in emergency for excessive bleeding during her heat cycle. She has free access to a large farm and piece of land. She has no prior illness history.

As her owner brings her to the clinic, Molly collapses in the parking lot, so she is rushed into the treatment area. Initial triage examination shows white mucous membranes with a very prolonged capillary refill time, weak pulses with a heart rate of 160 bpm, and cold extremities. She has obvious blood coming from her vulvar area. She is breathing rapidly but seems to have minimal distress. However, she has a fluid wave on abdominal palpation.

An intravenous catheter is placed, and a minimal database performed, including PCV-TP, a lactate level, an ECG and a blood pressure. PCV is 27% and TP is 4.1 g/dl, lactate is 7.6 mmol/l, ECG reveals a sinus tachycardia, and a Doppler blood pressure is 100 mm Hg. Upon questioning, the owner reveals that anticoagulant rodenticide is present in multiple areas of the barn. Point-of-care ultrasound confirms the presence of abdominal effusion, which is diagnosed as a hemoabdomen upon abdominocentesis.

Suspecting a coagulopathy secondary to anticoagulant rodenticide toxicity, the clinician orders a full blood work, including PT/aPTT, as well as a complete blood count, a biochemistry profile, and a blood type. Without knowing the results, the clinician also asks for fresh frozen plasma to be thawed.

Estimating the dog's body weight to be 20 kg, we would recommend using at least plasma at 10 ml/kg, but probably closer to 15–20 ml/kg for this specific patient, as she is experiencing severe hemorrhagic shock. Fresh frozen plasma, frozen plasma and cryo-poor plasma can be used in this indication, as these all contain the vitamin K-dependent factors (II, VII, IX, X). As most units of FFP are 200 ml/kg, we would provide 2 units of plasma products.

Due to the emergency situation, minimal isotonic crystalloids should be provided (a 10 ml/kg bolus over 20 min is reasonable while the plasma is thawing (see Chapter 6.i for rationale) and the plasma product should be "flash-thawed" using a warm running-water bath, which takes approximately 15 min. After thawing, the plasma product is administered as a bolus, providing both intravascular blood volume for shock resuscitation as well as coagulation factors, with 400 ml (20 ml/kg) over 20–30 min.

Because the patient is anemic, Molly can be provided with a packed red blood cell transfusion (pRBC), or an autotransfusion can also be performed if no pRBC is available or if finances are limited.

Clinical Case 4ii.2

Brutus is a 5-year-old castrated male Golden Retriever (28 kg), who is recovering from a jejunal resection and anastomosis following intestinal perforation due to a foreign body obstruction and septic peritonitis. For the purpose of the case example, the relevant information is that the albumin concentration is 2.1 g/dl, the Jackson-Pratt drain production is moderate to marked, and the mean arterial blood pressure measured with a direct arterial blood pressure catheter placed during anesthesia is hovering around 65 mm Hg.

Use of albumin in this indication is controversial. What we know in veterinary medicine is that hypoalbuminemia carries a worse prognosis and that albumin replacement using canine plasma product will raise the albumin level. However, it is unclear if providing albumin replacement will improve mortality in veterinary patients or people. As this dog is potentially going into septic shock, albumin replacement makes physiological sense. Due to the risk associated with human serum albumin, a canine-specific plasma product is recommended. Because the origin of the calculation and replacement of the albumin deficit commonly used in veterinary medicine is probably not applicable to critically ill dogs, we would use a fixed dose of albumin.

Although CPP has a higher albumin content than FFP, the difference is unlikely to be clinically significant and FFP is more commonly used. Instead, the target will be to provide 1 g/kg/day, which is a commonly used dosage of albumin in people in septic shock. To determine the hourly rate of infusion:

$$(1\text{g}/\text{kg}/\text{day})/24\text{h} = 0.042\text{g}/\text{kg}/\text{h} \times 1000\text{mg}/\text{g} = 42\text{mg}/\text{kg}/\text{h}$$

$$\text{Albumin concentration ofFFP} = (2.9\text{g}/\text{dl} \times 1000\text{mg}/\text{g})/(100\text{ml}/\text{dl}) = 29\text{mg}/\text{ml}$$

$$(40\text{mg}/\text{kg}/\text{h})/(29\text{mg}/\text{ml}) = 1.7\text{ml}/\text{kg}/\text{h}$$

Therefore, we will provide canine-specific albumin replacement by starting Brutus on FFP at 1.7 ml/kg/h. This will result in administration of FFP at 48 ml/h, or 1.1 l/day.

References

Adamantos, S., Chan, D.L., Goggs, R. *et al.* (2009) Risk of immunologic reactions to human serum albumin solutions. *Journal of Small Animal Practice* 50, 206.

American Thoracic Society (2004) Evidence-based colloid use in the critically ill: American Thoracic Society Consensus Statement. *American Journal of Respiratory Critical Care Medicine* 170, 1247–1259.

Boldt, J. (2010) Use of albumin: an update. *British Journal of Anaesthesiology* 104, 276–284.

Brown, R.O., Bradley, J.E. and Luther, R.W. (1987) Response of serum albumin concentrations to albumin supplementation during central total parenteral nutrition. *Clinical Pharmacology* 6, 222–226.

Caironi, P., Tognoni, G., Masson, S. *et al.* (2014). Albumin replacement in patients with severe sepsis or septic shock. *New England Journal of Medicine* 370, 1412–1421.

Chan, DL. (2008) Colloids: current recommendations. *Veterinary Clinics of North America Small Animal Practice* 38, 587–593.

Craft, E.M. and Powell, L.L. (2012) The use of canine-specific albumin in dogs with septic peritonitis. *Journal of Veterinary Emergency and Critical Care* 22, 631–639.

Culler, C.A., Iazbik, C. and Guillaumin, J. (2017) Comparison of albumin, colloid osmotic pressure, von Willebrand factor, and coagulation factors in canine cryopoor plasma, cryoprecipitate, and fresh frozen plasma. *Journal of Veterinary Emergency and Critical Care* 27, 638–644.

Culler, C.A., Balakrishnan, A., Yaxley, P.E. *et al.* (2019) Clinical use of cryopoor plasma continuous rate infusion in critically ill, hypoalbuminemic dogs. *Journal of Veterinary Emergency and Critical Care* 29, 314–320.

Davidow, B. (2013) Transfusion medicine in small animals. *Veterinary Clinics of North America Small Animal Practice* 43, 735–756.

Ewalenko, P., Deloof, T. and Peeters. J. (1986) Composition of fresh frozen plasma. *Critical Care Medicine* 14, 145–146.

Francis, A.H., Martin, L.G., Haldorson, G.J. *et al.* (2007) Adverse reactions suggestive of type III hypersensitivity in six healthy dogs given human albumin. *Journal of the American Veterinary Medical Association* 230, 873–879.

Grochowsky, A.R., Rozanski, E.A., de Laforcade, A.M. *et al.* (2014). An ex vivo evaluation of efficacy of refrigerated canine plasma. *Journal of Veterinary Emergency and Critical Care* 24, 388–397.

Hurst, T.S., Turrentine, M.A. and Johnson, G.S. (1987) Evaluation of microwave-thawed canine plasma for transfusion. *Journal of the American Veterinary Medical Association* 190, 863–865.

Powell, C., Thompson, L. and Murtaugh, R.J. (2013) Type III hypersensitivity reaction with immune complex deposition in 2 critically ill dogs administered human serum albumin. *Journal of Veterinary Emergency and Critical Care* 23, 598–604.

Roberts, I., Blackhall, K., Alderson, P. *et al.* (2011) Human albumin solution for resuscitation and volume expansion in critically ill patients. *Cochrane Database of Systematic Reviews* 2011(11), CD001208.

Ropski, M.K., Guillaumin, J., Monnig, A.A. *et al.* (2017) Use of cryopoor plasma for albumin replacement and continuous antimicrobial infusion for treatment of septic peritonitis in a dog. *Journal of Veterinary Emergency and Critical Care* 27, 348–356.

Roux, F., Deswarte, A. and Deschamps, J. (2013) Prognostic value of preoperative serum albumin level in canine and feline gastro-intestinal surgery: 150 cases (2009–2012). *Journal of Veterinary Emergency and Critical Care* 23, S17.

Rozanski, E.A., Hughes, D. and Giger, U. (2001) The effect of heparin and fresh frozen plasma on plasma antithrombin III activity, prothrombin time and activated partial thromboplastin time in critically ill dogs. *Journal of Veterinary Emergency and Critical Care* 11, 15–21.

Rozga, J., Piątek, T. and Małkowski, P. (2013) Human albumin: old, new, and emerging applications. *Annals of Transplant* 18, 205–217.

SAFE Study Investigators (2011) Impact of albumin compared to saline on organ function and mortality of patients with severe sepsis. *Intensive Care Medicine* 37, 86–96.

Sihler, K.C. and Napolitano, L.M. (2009) Massive transfusion: new insights. *Chest* 136, 1654–1667.

Snow, S.J., Jutkowitz, A.L. and Brown, A.J. (2010) Trends in plasma transfusion at a veterinary teaching hospital: 308 patients (1996–1998 and 2006–2008). *Journal of Veterinary Emergency and Critical Care* 20, 441–445.

Torkildsen, L., Bishop, M.A., Barr, J.W. *et al.* (2018) Comparison of multiple thawing techniques on thaw time and stability of hemostatic proteins in canine plasma products. *Journal of Small Animal Practice* 59, 641–645.

Trow, A.V., Rozanski, E.A., Delaforcade, A.M. *et al.* (2008) Evaluation of use of human albumin in critically ill dogs: 73 cases (2003-2006). *Journal of the American Veterinary Medical Association* 233, 607–612.

Turner, M.A., Rahilly, L.J. and O'Marra, K.S. (2018) Ex vivo evaluation of the efficacy of canine fresh-frozen plasma thawed using a microwave plasma defroster. *Journal of Veterinary Emergency and Critical Care* 28, 603–607.

Urban, R., Couto, G.C. and Iazbik, M.C. (2013) Evaluation of hemostatic activity of canine frozen plasma for transfusion by thromboelastography. *Journal of Veterinary Internal Medicine* 27, 964–969.

Viganó, F., Perissinotto, L. and Bosco, VR. (2010) Administration of 5% human serum albumin in critically ill small animal patients with hypoalbuminemia: 418 dogs and 170 cats (1994–2008). *Journal of Veterinary Emergency and Critical Care* 20, 237–243.

Vincent, J.L. (2009) Relevance of albumin in modern critical care medicine. *Best Practice and Research. Clinical Anaesthesiology* 23, 183–191.

5 Routes of Fluid Administration

EDWARD COOPER

The Ohio State University, Columbus, Ohio, USA

Now that the different types of fluids have been presented, the next major consideration in developing a fluid therapy plan is determining the optimal route of delivery. The goal of this chapter is not to provide a description of the technical aspects of establishing vascular access; the reader is directed to other resources if that information is needed (Burkett and Davis, 2012; Silverstein and Hopper, 2015). Instead, the purpose will be to provide guidance in deciding which route of delivery is best suited to the patient's needs. Several different routes of delivery will be explored, along with the factors that might impact which one is chosen, and the advantages and disadvantages of each.

5.1 Overview of Routes and Factors Affecting Selection

The main potential routes that can be utilized are summarized in Table 5.1. These include the intravenous (IV) route, which can be either central or peripheral, use of the intraosseous route (IO), subcutaneous administration (SC), or delivery using the enteral route (EN). Numerous factors can impact which of these are going to be the most appropriate for the individual patient (Table 5.1). A main consideration is the overall reason that fluids need to be administered. This can be best thought of from the standpoint of the different phases of fluid therapy: **resuscitation** (rapid expansion of vascular volume); **replacement** (of dehydration and ongoing losses); and **maintenance** (providing daily fluid needs). As will be discussed extensively in Chapter 6, each of these requires different rates and volumes to be administered. Along similar lines, the nature, severity, and acuity of the disease process will likely impact the fluid therapy plan and whether hospitalization versus outpatient care is warranted. For example, rapid, large volume, and/or ongoing fluid administration can be achieved better with some routes (e.g., IV and IO), but not others (e.g., SC and EN).

In addition to medical factors, sometimes practical or logistical considerations can affect which routes can be used. As previously discussed, the composition of some fluids is hypertonic or hypotonic, and may be irritating or harmful if given in a peripheral IV or in the SC space. Certain types of catheter (central IV or IO) require more technical expertise and previous experience in order to be placed. The required equipment is also needed (such as a central line or IO catheter), even if a member of the team is comfortable with placement. A final consideration, and potentially the most impactful on the decision of how to proceed, is whether the owner has the resources necessary for the ideal route and level of care. While hospitalization and IV fluids may be preferred by the practitioner, if the owner is unable to afford that treatment path a different route might have to be selected.

5.2 Intravenous Route

Obtaining IV access is the most utilized route for in-hospital fluid therapy, and overall offers the most versatility. With direct access to the vascular space there is the opportunity to deliver large volumes at a rapid rate. In this regard the IV route can be used for all phases of fluid administration. In addition, all types and categories of fluids can be given IV, including crystalloids, colloids, and blood products. Further, it is possible to give fluids that are significantly hypertonic or hypotonic, particularly if central access has been obtained. Aside from fluid therapy, IV access can also be used to administer any other injectable medications that are needed for patient management. For these reasons, the IV route is particularly preferred for fluid resuscitation, patients with significant dehydration and/or ongoing losses, patients undergoing general anesthesia,

DOI: 10.1079/9781789243406.0005

Table 5.1. Summary of available routes of delivery, and the factors that may play a role in deciding which to choose.

Routes of delivery	Factors affecting choice
Intravenous • Central or peripheral Intraosseus Subcutaneous Enteral	Purpose of fluid administration Nature of the clinical disorder • Acute versus chronic • Severity • Hospitalized versus outpatient care Nature and magnitude of ongoing losses Composition of fluid to be administered Technical expertise Equipment availability Owner financial capabilities

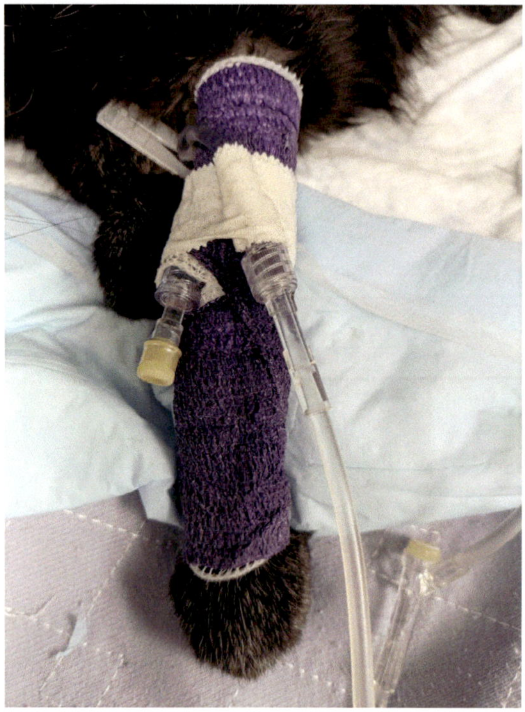

Fig. 5.1. Feline patient with a peripheral catheter in the left cephalic vein.

patients requiring hospitalization, and certainly any critically ill patient. Depending on patient needs and availability, IV access can be in the form of either a peripheral catheter or a central line.

5.2.1 Peripheral venous

Peripheral catheters are by far the more commonly used means of achieving IV access. These catheters are typically easier to place, as they require less technical expertise and specialized equipment compared with central lines. Care and maintenance are also generally less involved, and peripheral catheters are typically less expensive (though cost may become closer if there is a need to place several). There are some drawbacks to peripheral access. Depending on placement, these catheters can be positional and become occluded with limb movement (especially if placed too proximally). They can also be short-lived compared with central catheters. As they are placed in smaller veins, fluids that are hypotonic or hypertonic in nature are more likely to cause vessel irritation (phlebitis), especially if given as prolonged infusions (for example, total parenteral nutrition and solutions containing >5% dextrose).

There are many different sizes of peripheral catheter that can be placed, depending on the size of the patient and the target vessel. Catheters ranging from 18- to 22-gauge are most commonly used for small animal patients. That said, a large dog may be able to accommodate a 16-gauge catheter, and very small patients or pediatrics may need as small as 24-gauge. Vessel selection may also be important, and there can be some species variation. For both dogs and cats, the **forelimb cephalic vessel** can be a good option (Fig. 5.1), particularly for patients experiencing shock and needing fluid resuscitation. The cephalic vein, compared with more caudal vessels, is closer to the heart, and less likely to be affected by disease processes that may cause obstruction of venous return (such as gastric dilatation and volvulus). Along similar lines, a **peripheral catheter placed in the jugular vein** may be viable when cephalic access is unsuccessful (particularly in smaller patients and pediatrics). While this is still considered peripheral access, the large vessel size and proximity to the central compartment make this a good option in the crashing patient. For dogs, additional options for peripheral access include the **lateral saphenous vein** and the **dorsal pedal vein** (Fig. 5.2). The other main peripheral location for cats is the **medial saphenous**. The technical aspects of peripheral catheter placement and maintenance are beyond the intent of this chapter, and other resources are recommended (Davis, 2015a).

5.2.2 Central venous

By definition, central venous access reflects that the tip of the catheter is in a great vessel, like the caudal or cranial vena cava, or the main venous branches just prior. The most common site for introducing a central line is the jugular vein, though a peripheral vessel like the saphenous can be the access point as long as the catheter reaches a central vein (this is called a PICC, or **peripherally inserted central catheter**). There are several advantages to central line placement. Central catheters can be **single lumen** or **multi-lumen** (Fig. 5.3A), with the latter allowing for multiple dedicated infusions as the ports are kept separate the entire length (Fig. 5.3B). With access to a central vein, serial blood sampling can be performed through catheter, thereby reducing the need to perform repeated venipuncture (and associated stress). Significantly hypertonic or hypotonic fluids can be administered safely, and with proper maintenance central lines can remain in place for extended periods of time.

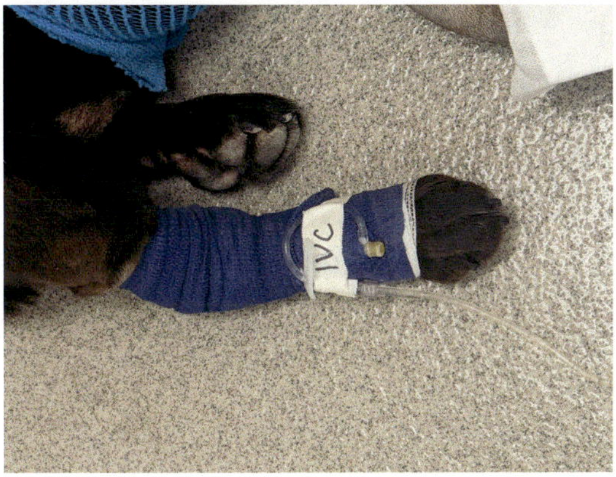

Fig. 5.2. Canine patient with a peripheral catheter in the dorsal pedal vein. Note: care has been taken to mark the catheter as IV to limit the chance of it being mistaken for a dorsal metatarsal arterial catheter, which would be in the same place.

Given the size of central lumen catheters, they are typically placed using the **Seldinger technique**. This entails placing an initial smaller introducing catheter, passing a guidewire to hold the vessel, and then using a dilator to allow the larger central catheter to be inserted and then secured. A more detailed description of the technique can be found elsewhere (Davis, 2015b). The more complex nature of central line placement is one of the main inherent limitations – they require a greater level of training and expertise, and have more associated cost, compared with peripheral catheter placement. In addition, all but the sickest of patients will typically require some measure of sedation to facilitate placement. Finally, using the jugular vein to introduce a central line would be relatively contraindicated in patients with bleeding disorders. In those circumstances, placement of a PICC would be safer if central access is needed.

5.2.3 Administration

Calculating the volume and rate of infusion will be discussed extensively in Chapter 6. Once these have

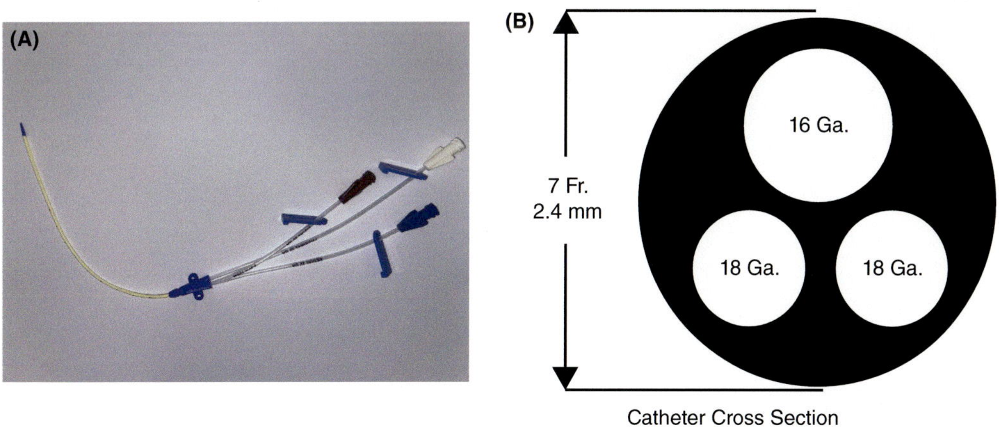

Fig. 5.3. Images demonstrating **(A)** a triple-lumen central catheter, and **(B)** the cross-sectional arrangement of the three distinct lumens. As demonstrated, a 7 Fr. catheter contains two 18-gauge and one 16-gauge ports.

been decided, IV fluid administration can be achieved in two ways: a gravity-fed system or using a metered fluid pump. With a gravity-fed (drip) system, the bag is kept elevated so that fluid moves into the vein due to gravity. Administration sets include a roller clamp that allows the tubing to be more open or closed to flow, thereby controlling the rate of administration. It is important to note that the flow rate can also be affected by the position of the patient, height of the bag, and kinking of the catheter. Movement of the patient can result in significant changes in flow rate, and so patients on a gravity-fed system must be monitored closely. With this system it is also necessary to calculate the drip rate based on the infusion set, as they can have different drops/ml (10 versus 60). This information is then used to determine the drip rate to achieve the desired infusion rate. See Clinical Case 5.1 for an example of how this is performed.

While the gravity-fed system can be used, whenever possible a metered fluid pump is preferred for administration of intravenous fluids because this will help ensure accuracy. Volumetric pumps (Fig. 5.4A) are most commonly used as they can be programmed to accurately deliver rates up to 1 l/h (typically well within the range of small-animal fluid rates). If the desired rate is greater than this upper limit (such as a fluid bolus administration to a large dog), it may be necessary to use a drip-set as described above with application of a pressure bag. It should also be noted that most volumetric pumps become less accurate at very low fluid rates

Clinical Case 5.1

Your 20 kg canine patient needs to undergo anesthesia, and you plan to have him on 5 ml/kg/h (so 100 ml/h) of an isotonic crystalloid for the duration. Your clinic has been very busy, and you are informed that you are out of metered fluid pumps. The decision is made to use a drip-set and gravity-fed administration. Here are the calculations for determining the drip rate:

$$100\ \text{ml/h} \times 1\ \text{h}/60\ \text{min} = 1.67\ \text{ml/min} \times 1\text{min}/60\ \text{sec} = 0.02\ \text{ml/sec}$$

$$0.02\ \text{ml/sec} \times 10\ \text{drops/ml} = 0.2\ \text{drops/sec} = 1\ \text{drop every 5 seconds}$$

In this circumstance, the drip rate would be adjusted until one drop every 5 seconds is achieved. Thankfully as the patient is under general anesthesia changes in rate secondary to movement are unlikely to occur. However, the drip rate is still reassessed frequently to ensure it is still one drop per 5 seconds.

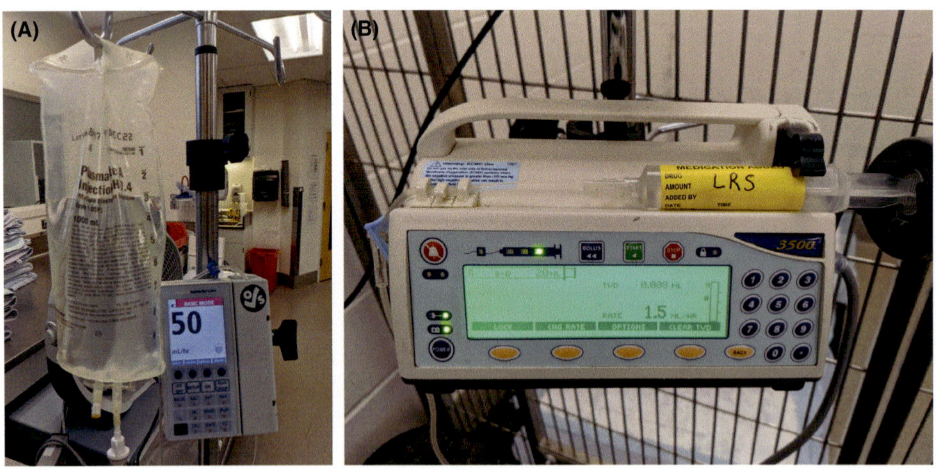

Fig. 5.4. Examples of **(A)** a volumetric pump and **(B)** a syringe pump.

(especially <2 ml/h). In these circumstances it may be better to use a syringe pump, as they are typically metered to run at much lower rates (Fig. 5.4B).

5.2.4 Complications

While there are lots of benefits associated with having intravenous access, some complications can arise. There is potential for extravasation of the catheter to occur (particularly peripheral), resulting in subcutaneous administration of fluids and medications. Depending on the volume and nature of the material, this could result in swelling, erythema, and/or significant tissue damage. Thrombophlebitis and thrombosis are also potential complications, with the latter having the potential for significant concern (like a pulmonary thromboembolism). Finally, there is potential for catheter-site, or catheter-associated (bloodstream) infections.

5.3 Intraosseous Route

In circumstances where IV access is needed but cannot be achieved, IO catheter placement may offer a viable alternative. Most often this would be in circumstances of cardiovascular collapse or cardiac arrest (such that the veins are too collapsed to find or catheterize), or in very small patients like neonates and pediatrics (such that the veins are too small to accommodate a catheter). The medullary cavity does not collapse in hypovolemia and may more readily accommodate catheter placement compared with a peripheral vessel. In addition, instillation into the marrow cavity results in rapid redistribution to the vascular compartment. It is essentially the same as IV access, such that anything that is given IV can be given IO. In this regard, the acute applications for IO access are the same as mentioned above for IV, just reserved for when placing an IV catheter is not possible.

Several different catheter types can be used. These include commercially available IO needles, bone marrow needles, spinal needles, or hypodermic needles. The commercially available IO needles have the benefit of a powered drill, which can allow very rapid placement (Fig. 5.5). Selection depends on the size of the patient, available resources, and the intended location for placement. Most common sites include the greater tubercle of the humerus (Fig. 5.6), trochanteric fossa of the femur, tibial tuberosity, or wing of the ilium. The combination of a hypodermic needle into the trochanteric fossa works well for neonates/pediatrics, whereas IO or bone marrow needles into the humerus is the favored site for adult patients. A more detailed description of the technique for IO catheter placement can be found elsewhere (Giunti and Otto, 2015).

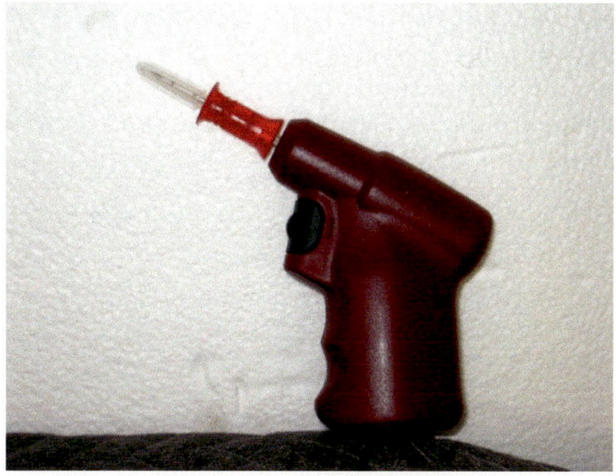

Fig. 5.5. A commercially available needle and drill system to facilitate obtaining IO access.

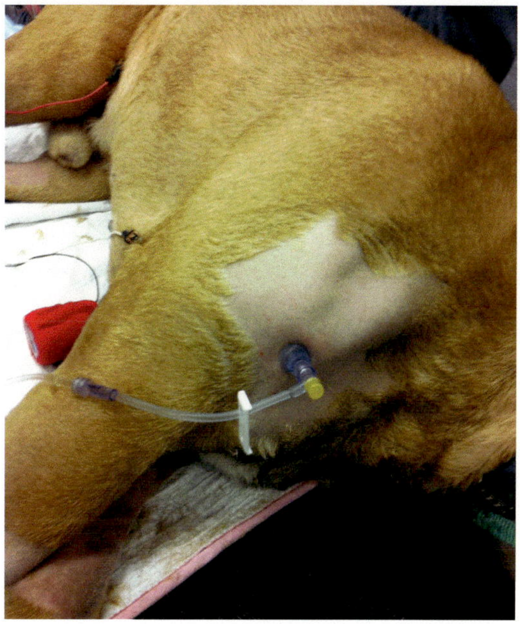

Fig. 5.6. Placement of an IO needle into the greater tubercle of the humerus in a dog.

5.3.1 Complications

While IO catheter placement can allow for rapid and effective access for fluid administration, there are some potential disadvantages. There can be a steep learning curve for the placement technique and ensuring that the marrow cavity has been achieved. Securing the needle can also be challenging, and IO access tends to be short-lived. Every opportunity should be made to obtain IV access once the patient is more stable and has been volume resuscitated. There is also the potential to introduce an infection at the time of placement, with development of osteomyelitis.

5.4 Subcutaneous Route

The SC route is another option for delivering fluids. The principle is that instillation of fluid into the SC space can serve as a repository and allow gradual absorption with subsequent redistribution over the span of (typically) 6–8 h. Use of the SC route carries the benefits of minimal cost, minimal equipment or expertise required, and the ability to manage outpatients (with owners potentially administering fluids at home). However, the rate of absorption will be impacted by hydration status, peripheral perfusion, and body temperature. With this in mind, it stands to reason that subcutaneous fluids will not be very effective in the face of severe dehydration, major electrolyte/metabolic abnormalities, hypovolemia, hypothermia and/or shock. This route is best applied to patients that can be treated on an outpatient basis with mild to moderate dehydration, patients that are euhydrated with decreased intake (to prevent dehydration), or in anticipation of increased losses. Use of SC fluid administration may also be necessary in circumstances whereby hospitalization and IV fluid therapy would be preferred, but the owners are unwilling or unable to do so.

5.4.1 Administration

Definitive guidelines for dosing SC fluids are lacking, and recommendations are largely based on clinical experience and "ball-park" estimates; for example, cats and small dogs 50–100 ml, medium dogs 250–500 ml, and large dogs 500–1000 ml. There are sometimes practical limitations relative to the amount of fluid that can safely be placed in the SC without risk of harm, and so this may also factor into the decision of how much to give. More precise calculations would involve trying to anticipate daily fluid needs (maintenance) as well as addressing dehydration (replacement). See Clinical Case 5.2 for example calculations that demonstrate the potential volumes that would come about from this process. Based on those calculations, the 5 kg feline patient would potentially need 600 ml of fluid. While this is completely impractical, it also becomes clear how relatively little contribution the "ball-park" dose of 50–100 ml would provide for this patient. So how, then, should SC fluid be dosed? Provided there are no specific contraindications (such as known underlying heart disease), targeting 20–30 ml/kg (or about half of daily maintenance requirement) is a reasonable starting point. To facilitate administration of larger volumes, it may be helpful to use a pressure bag to decrease delivery time (Fig. 5.7). If deemed necessary, the owner is willing, and the patient is tolerant, additional doses could be given every 12 h.

Another consideration is what type of fluid to use. To minimize the risk of irritation or tissue damage, isotonic fluids like 0.9% NaCl or LRS should be used. Previously, Plasma-Lyte was avoided as the more acidic version (Plasma-Lyte 148) could cause discomfort when given SC.

Clinical Case 5.2

A 5 kg FS DSH cat presents for vomiting and anorexia. She is determined to be 7% dehydrated, but otherwise vitals are normal and there are no other obvious abnormalities on physical examination. Radiographs reveal no evidence of mechanical obstruction, and blood work is relatively unremarkable aside from an increase in PCV/TP (fitting with dehydration). Hospitalization for rehydration and supportive care is offered, but the owner elects outpatient management. You determine her daily maintenance fluid requirement and replacement of dehydration over 24 h (see Chapters 6ii and 6iii for more information on these calculations):

$$\text{Daily maintenance} = 80 \times \text{wt}^{0.75} = 80 \times 5^{0.75} = 260 \text{ ml}$$

$$\text{Replacement} = 5 \text{ kg} \times 0.07 = 350 \text{ ml}$$

$$\text{Total volume to administer} = 350 \text{ ml} + 260 \text{ ml} = 610 \text{ ml}$$

Obviously, this would be far too large a volume to administer SC. A target of trying to provide half the maintenance or replacement volumes would be a reasonable place to start, 20–30 ml/kg, or 100–150 ml. If the owner is comfortable doing so, they could give additional doses at home.

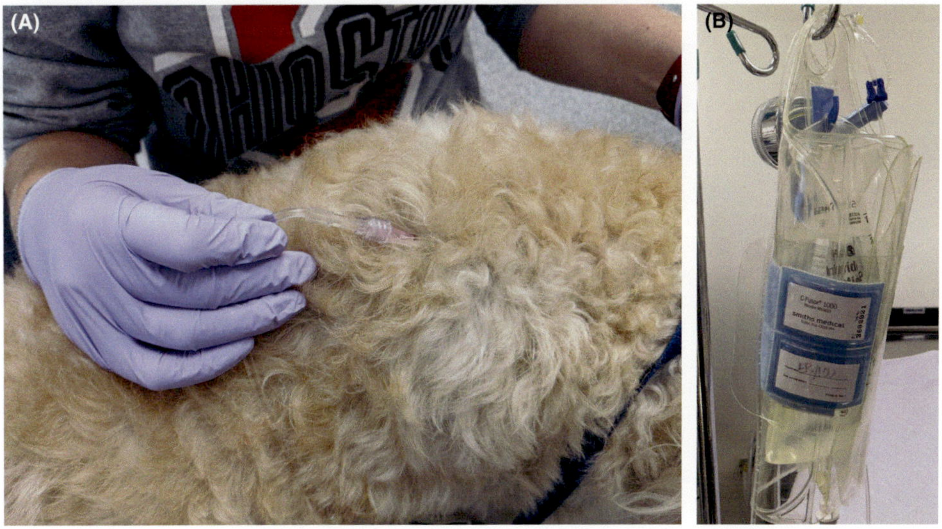

Fig. 5.7. Canine patient receiving SC fluids **(A)** with a pressure bag used to facilitate delivery **(B)**.

However, this appears to be less of a concern with the neutral Plasma-Lyte A. Dextrose solutions containing a concentration greater than 2.5% should not be given SC, as there is potential to cause necrosis and abscess formation.

5.4.2 Complications

While administration of SC may have application in some patients, there are potential complications that can arise. If too much fluid is delivered in one location, the associated pressure can cause some of the fluid to leak back out (making it less effective). Excessive pressure can also cause pain and irritation, with the potential to result in necrosis. During administration it is important to palpate the area to ensure it is not becoming to firm. Dividing the target volume over multiple sites can also help limit this effect. Though the risk is very low, it is possible to introduce bacteria during this process and set the stage for cellulitis or abscess formation. Similarly, SC fluid administration to a patient with a bleeding disorder can lead to a hematoma formation.

5.5 Enteral route

The enteral route potentially constitutes the most natural way to provide daily water needs, as absorption through the GI tract is how intake occurs in health. Offering water to patients that have an intact thirst mechanism and functional gastrointestinal system can even preclude the need for IV fluid administration (as not every hospitalized patient needs to be on fluids!). If the primary issue is the drive to drink, patients with a feeding tube in place (e.g., nasogastric or esophagostomy) offer a good opportunity to provide enteral water while in hospital and lessen the amount of intravenous fluids administered. This could be particularly important in patients that may be less tolerant of sodium load, such as those with cardiac or kidney disease (see Chapters 8iii and 8iv). After calculation of the maintenance fluid requirement (see Chapter 6iii), it can be determined what portion can be delivered by the enteral route.

However, there are several circumstances whereby the enteral route might not be ideal. This would be particularly the case for any patients with significant primary GI disease, or that are cardiovascularly unstable. In the face of hypovolemia and hypotension, GI perfusion and thereby absorption will be limited, and enteral water will only contribute to distention and gastric residuals. In addition, for patients with severe dehydration and/or significant ongoing losses, it may be difficult to provide a sufficient quantity of fluid to meet the patient's needs. If the deficit or losses are isotonic in nature, then replacing only water may not be sufficient, and electrolyte depletion could occur. In these circumstances, using an oral solution containing electrolytes may be of benefit.

Enteral fluids can also be used for at-home management for patients with feeding tubes in place,

Table 5.2. Summary overview of benefits and limitations of various routes of administration.

Route	Advantages/indications	Disadvantages
IV	Direct access to vascular volume Administer large volumes rapidly Can use multiple fluid types All phases of fluid therapy	Catheter problems Cost/technical limitations Risk of thrombosis/phlebitis Risk of infection
IO	Alternative to IV access • Cardiovascular collapse/arrest • Neonates and pediatric	Can be technically challenging Risk of infection/hematoma Short-term option
SC	Ease Minimal cost Outpatient use Mild/moderate dehydration	Cannot give large volumes Slow transfer to other compartments Isotonic fluids only Should not be used in shock
EN	Ease Non-sterile Outpatient use with feeding tube	Need functional GI May not be able to provide enough volume Should not be used in shock

such as esophagostomy or gastrostomy tubes. For example, patients with chronic kidney disease can have difficulty maintaining hydration in the face of polyuria and decreased drinking. While this is often managed with intermittent SC fluid administration by owners, enteral water through a feeding tube may be preferable and better tolerated. As previously indicated, enteral water provides a more physiological source of hydration and does not contain the unneeded additional sodium burden of isotonic crystalloids.

5.6 Summary

Ultimately, selection of the route of admission is dependent on a number of factors, as outlined in this chapter. Table 5.2 provides a summary of the potential applications and indications for each route, as well as some of the disadvantages and contraindications.

References

Burkett, J.M. and Davis, H. (2012) *Advanced Monitoring and Procedures for Small Animal Emergency and Critical Care*, 1st edn. John Wiley and Sons, Ames, Iowa.

Davis, H. (2015a) Peripheral venous catheterization. In: Silverstein, D.C. and Hopper, K. (eds) *Small Animal Critical Care Medicine*, 2nd edn. Elsevier, Amsterdam, Netherlands, pp. 1005–1008.

Davis, H. (2015b) Central venous catheterization. In: Silverstein, D.C. and Hopper, K. (eds) *Small Animal Critical Care Medicine*, 2nd edn. Elsevier, Amsterdam, Netherlands, pp. 1013–1017.

Giunti, M. and Otto, C.M. (2015) Intraosseous catheterization. In: Silverstein, D.C. and Hopper, K. (eds) *Small Animal Critical Care Medicine*, 2nd edn. Elsevier, Amsterdam, Netherlands, pp. 1009–1013.

Silverstein, D.C. and Hopper, K. (eds) (2015) *Small Animal Critical Care Medicine*, 2nd edn. Elsevier, Amsterdam, Netherlands.

6i Resuscitation Fluid Therapy

EDWARD COOPER

The Ohio State University, Columbus, Ohio, USA

Now that the concepts of fluid type and route of delivery have been considered, it is time to move on to the remaining cardinal questions of fluid therapy: how much and how fast? To answer these questions, it is important to consider the goal of fluid administration for the individual patient. For example, a patient in shock might require acute expansion of the vascular volume (**resuscitation**), whereas another patient might need more gradual administration of fluids to address dehydration and ongoing loses (**replacement**), and yet another may only need provision of daily fluid requirement (**maintenance**). The clinical situation and patient assessment serve to indicate which of these best fits the patient's needs. The three sections of this 'General Approach to Fluid Therapy' chapter (6i, 6ii, and 6iii) will provide a framework for the general approach to each phase of fluid therapy, including recognition, guidelines for fluid administration, and monitoring.

6i.1 Indications for Resuscitation Fluid Therapy

As previously indicated, the goal of fluid resuscitation is focused on expansion of the vascular compartment in order to address a decrease in absolute or effective circulating volume that has resulted in cardiovascular compromise (shock). A complete description of the different causes of shock and associated pathogenesis is beyond the scope of this chapter, but is available in other resources (Muir, 2006; Cooper, 2019). A brief overview will be provided here in the context of fluid resuscitation.

6i.1.1 Causes of shock

In its broadest sense, **shock** is any circumstance whereby metabolic demand for oxygen exceeds uptake and utilization. The result is the development of cellular energy debt and dysfunction, ultimately progressing to organ failure, cardiovascular collapse, and death of the patient despite compensatory efforts. Therefore, early recognition and intervention to reverse the shock state are essential for patient survival. Multiple categorical schemes have been developed based on the underlying mechanism for the development of shock (Table 6i.1) and ultimately relate to the major factors that contribute to normal cardiovascular homeostasis (see the "tree of life" in Fig. 6i.1).

With regard to shock resuscitation, the unifying theme for when a patient may be fluid responsive is in circumstances when preload is reduced (Table 6i.1). **Preload** is a term used to reflect stretching of the ventricle prior to contraction and is largely dictated by venous return. As such, an increase in preload is associated with an increase in stroke volume and cardiac output (direct relationship), with the reverse also being true (a decrease in preload will decrease stroke volume). Hypovolemic, obstructive, and maldistributive causes of shock are all associated with a decrease in preload. In the case of **hypovolemia**, there is an absolute reduction of circulating volume leading to decreased venous return (e.g., hemorrhage). With **obstructive shock**, a normal volume may be present, but it is trapped behind some obstruction to venous return (e.g., GDV). In **maldistributive shock** (e.g., sepsis) there is inappropriate vasodilation. On the arterial side it makes intuitive sense that this will result in a decrease in systemic vascular resistance and negatively impact blood pressure. However, it may be less intuitive that relaxation of veins can serve to markedly increase their capacity to hold volume. As a result of making the "tank" bigger, a normal amount of volume is now associated with a decreased venous return and preload. It then becomes evident that fluid administration can be beneficial in these clinical circumstances (along

DOI: 10.1079/9781789243406.0061

Table 6i.1. Categorical causes of shock with selected examples.

Categorical cause	Mechanism of shock	Examples	Fluid responsive?
Hypovolemia	Absolute ↓ preload	Hemorrhage Severe dehydration	Yes
Obstructive	Relative ↓ preload	GDV Pericardial effusion	Yes
Maldistributive	Relative ↓ preload ↓ SVR	Sepsis Anaphylaxis	Yes
Cardiogenic	↓ Contractility ↓ or ↑ in HR	Cardiomyopathy Severe tachy/bradyarrhythmia	No
Anemia/hypoxemia	↓ CaO_2	Hemolytic anemia Severe pulmonary dysfunction	No
Metabolic	Failure of cellular energy production	Hypoglycemia Sepsis	Maybe

CaO_2, arterial oxygen content; GDV, gastric dilatation and volvulus; HR, heart rate; SVR, systemic vascular resistance

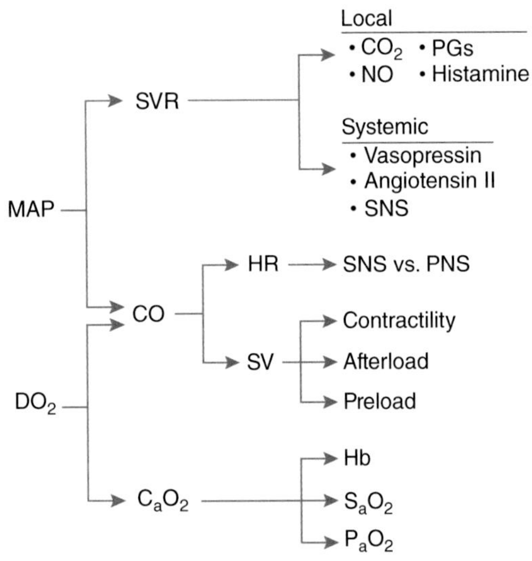

Fig. 6i.1. The "tree of life", representing the key physiologic factors that determine mean arterial pressure and oxygen delivery. CaO_2, arterial oxygen content; CO, cardiac output; CO_2, carbon dioxide; DO_2, oxygen delivery; Hb, hemoglobin; HR, heart rate; MAP, mean arterial pressure; NO, nitric oxide; PaO_2, partial pressure of oxygen; PGs, prostaglandins; PNS, parasympathetic nervous system; SaO_2, hemoglobin oxygen saturation; SNS, sympathetic nervous system; SV, stroke volume; SVR, systemic vascular resistance

with addressing the underlying cause) by promoting venous return, and thereby improving preload.

There are also circumstances of shock for which fluid therapy might not be beneficial or could even be harmful. This would most notably be the case with **cardiogenic shock**. These patients are typically experiencing decreased contractility, severe valvular regurgitation, and/or severe tachycardia/bradycardia. Further, these patients may have an increase in preload from fluid retention and be in or at risk of congestive heart failure. As such, volume loading and further increasing preload will not be helpful. True **anemic shock** is most often secondary to a hemolytic process (such as immune-mediated hemolytic anemia) or decreased production, rather than acute hemorrhage (where the shock is typically caused by hypovolemia, not anemia). These patients are more typically euvolemic (as only red blood cells have been lost) and therefore are best served receiving a red blood cell transfusion rather than crystalloids or colloids (unless concurrently dehydrated). **Hypoxemic shock** should be addressed by provision of supplemental oxygen or potentially mechanical ventilation, as there is no contribution of preload. For **metabolic shock**, it may depend on the cause. Hypoglycemia requires dextrose supplementation, and fluid administration may not be directly helpful. However, sepsis can be associated with mitochondrial dysfunction and fluids may play a role as described above.

While these concepts may seem relatively straightforward, part of the challenge may be that the underlying cause may not be evident at the time of shock recognition. Though it will be important to gather diagnostic information, there also should not be a delay in initiating resuscitative efforts. As described above, the longer that a patient is in shock, the greater is the damage that can occur and the harder it will be to achieve successful resuscitation/survival. The question then arises: without any other information, should the patient in shock

Table 6i.2. Expected changes in perfusion parameters relative to stage of shock.

	Compensated	Decompensated	Terminal
Mentation	Normal to quiet	Dull	Stupor to coma
Heart rate	Increased	Increased (cats maybe decreased)	Decreased
Mucous membranes	Pale pink	Pale	White
Capillary refill time	2–3 seconds	>3 seconds	Undetectable
Pulse quality	Moderate	Decreased	Absent
Extremity temperature	Normal to cool	Cool to cold	Cold

receive fluids while information is being gathered? Playing the odds, the answer is a resounding yes! As the fluid-responsive causes of shock tend to be more common (especially hypovolemia), it is reasonable to start resuscitation unless there is a clear contra-indication (such as known heart disease).

6i.1.2 Clinical signs of shock

Given the previous discussion, it stands to reason that recognition of shock is the most important aspect in deciding whether to initiate resuscitation fluid therapy. This determination is often made through a combination of clinical history and triage/physical examination. In conjunction with these, additional diagnostics can also be helpful to characterize the severity of shock, as well as determine the underlying cause (Table 6i.2).

Clinical history can help to raise the concern for circumstances associated with causing a shock state. Owners may report a recent traumatic event, collapsing episode, loss of consciousness, acute abdominal distention, pallor, etc. In addition, the triage assessment/physical examination should be the strongest initial indication of cardiovascular compromise and will be impacted by the stage of shock (Table 6i.2). These stages are reflective of the body's effort to maintain homeostasis (**compensated**), which can be subsequently overwhelmed (**decompensated**), and eventually become exhausted (**terminal**). The compensatory efforts are mediated predominantly through compartmental fluid shifts and the sympathetic nervous system initially, with additional support from the renin–angiotensin–aldosterone system and release of vasopressin/anti-diuretic hormone. These function to increase circulating volume, increase heart rate and contractility, and promote peripheral vasoconstriction, all in an effort to maintain core perfusion pressure (mean arterial pressure). As such, these compensatory efforts also create most of the outward manifestations

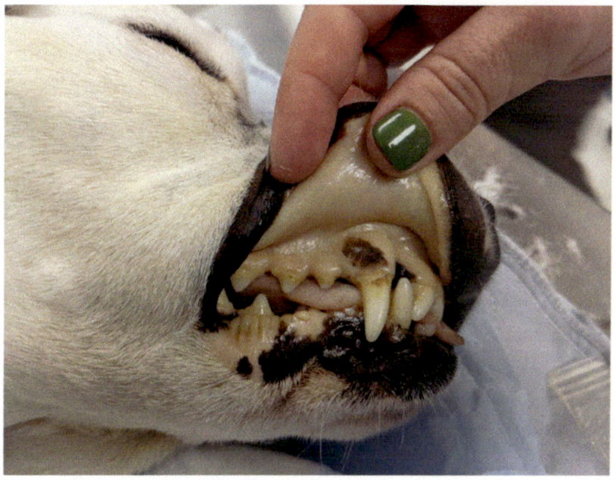

Fig. 6i.2. A canine patient with severe pallor associated with shock and hypoperfusion.

of shock as reflected by the six "perfusion parameters" (Table 6i.2, Fig. 6i.2). The progression to **decompensated shock** is characterized by the development of hypotension and a decrease in core perfusion. This is associated with a worsening of perfusion parameters, particularly a decline in mentation. Cats may become bradycardic at this stage. With **terminal shock** the compensatory efforts have become exhausted secondary to hyporeactivity and prolonged acidosis. At this point bradycardia, vasodilation, and venous pooling predominate with (as the name would imply) imminent cardiac arrest.

After physical examination, an **electrocardiogram** (ECG) offers important information in the assessment of a patient in shock. Typically quick and easy to apply, it can provide continuous information regarding heart rate and response to fluid resuscitation. Further, ECG allows assessment of any cardiac arrhythmias that may warrant treatment. The next most important piece of information is **blood pressure**. However, it is important to note that obtaining a blood pressure reading should not be necessary to determine if a patient is in shock, and fluid administration should not be delayed waiting for that information. This is especially true given that blood pressure can be challenging to obtain, especially in the face of hypotension. It is also important to note that a normal blood pressure does not guarantee cardiovascular stability: a patient can still be in (compensated) shock. As previously indicated, maintaining blood pressure is the purpose of the compensatory system and so it is the last thing to go. Said another way, a low blood pressure reading is bad, but a normal one does not mean the patient is cardiovascularly stable! However, once hypotension develops, the patient has progressed to decompensation and this can be important information to have. Obtaining a baseline blood pressure is also a key component of monitoring response to therapy. Full consideration of the techniques, benefits and drawbacks to modalities for monitoring blood pressure is beyond the scope of this chapter and can be found elsewhere (Williamson and Leone, 2012; Waddell and Brown, 2015).

As both heart rate and blood pressure can be impacted by other physiological stimuli (e.g., pain and stress), combining them to determine a **shock index** can also be beneficial. This is achieved by dividing the heart rate by the systolic blood pressure (HR/SBP). Shock index values >1.0 may be more reflective of a shock state warranting fluid resuscitation (Peterson *et al.*, 2013; Porter *et al.*, 2013).

There are additional diagnostics that may be of benefit in helping to guide fluid therapy for the patient in shock, as well as helping to determine the underlying cause (Box 6i.1).

Packed cell volume and total protein (PCV/TP) can offer important insight regarding the presence and severity of dehydration (typically an increase in both), loss of protein-rich fluid (PCV increased, TP normal to low), or the presence of hemorrhage (both decreased). It is important to note that with acute hemorrhage (within 30–60 min), a decrease in TP might be seen first, as splenic contraction sustains the PCV for longer. Blood lactate levels, as a marker for anaerobic metabolism, can be helpful to gauge severity of shock and in monitoring response to therapy. And while the initial value is important, how the lactate changes in response to therapy is likely much more important (Rosenstein *et al.*, 2018). Additional *statim* (stat) blood work may provide assessment of acid–base status, as well as indicate the presence of electrolyte abnormalities and/or azotemia. Obtaining a urine sample to determine specific gravity can be helpful in distinguishing pre-renal from renal azotemia. Ideally this is done as early into fluid therapy as possible, so as not to obscure the ability to make that determination. Perhaps one of the most powerful bedside tools to gather additional information regarding the cause of shock is the use of point-of-care ultrasound (POCUS). Various techniques have been described (Lisciandro and Lisciandro, 2021) and complete discussion is beyond the scope of this chapter. Briefly, POCUS can help to identify the presence of cavitary fluid (pleural, peritoneal or pericardial) or pneumothrorax, evidence of pulmonary pathology, and offer subjective assessment of volume status and cardiac function. If cavitary fluid is identified, preforming a diagnostic or therapeutic centesis is essential to support the patient and characterize the nature of the effusion (hemorrhage versus septic effusion versus neoplastic, etc). After initial stabilization, further diagnostics may include abdominal and/or thoracic radiographs, full abdominal ultrasound or CT, complete systemic blood work, coagulation testing, etc.

Box 6i.1. Point-of-care diagnostics that can be helpful in shock assessment and monitoring.

- ECG
- Blood pressure
- Packed cell volume/total protein
- Lactate
- Stat blood panel (acid–base and electrolytes)
- Blood urea nitrogen/creatinine
- Urine specific gravity
- Point-of-care ultrasound

6i.2 What type? Fluids Used in Resuscitation

There has been extensive experimental and clinical investigation in both human and veterinary medicine to determine the optimal type of fluid to use in resuscitation. Given the variety of clinical circumstances that can lead to shock and the need for acute volume expansion, it seems understandable that there is not one fluid type that is the clear victor. As discussed in Chapters 3 and 4, there are benefits and drawbacks to each different type of fluid. In this section they will be discussed briefly and specifically in the context of their application during fluid resuscitation. See Table 6i.3 for overarching recommendations.

6i.2.1 Hypotonic crystalloids

Hypotonic crystalloids (e.g., 0.45% NaCl, 5% dextrose in water, and Normosol M) have an osmolality less than that of blood, and so the volume of distribution is the total body water. As a result, only a very small portion of the volume administered will remain in the vascular space. In this regard they are very inefficient and ineffective at providing the acute volume expansion needed for resuscitation. In addition, rapid administration of hypotonic fluids could be harmful by causing sudden changes in blood osmolarity. The resulting osmotic injury is most impactful to red blood cells, vascular endothelium, and neuronal tissue. For all these reasons, hypotonic fluids should *not* be used for fluid resuscitation.

6i.2.2 Isotonic crystalloids

Isotonic crystalloids are the mainstay for fluid resuscitation, largely related to availability, versatility, and low cost associated with use. The volume of distribution for isotonic crystalloids is the extracellular space, meaning that with intravascular administration the majority will end up in the interstitial space (approximately two-thirds to three-quarters). As a result, a relatively large volume must be administered to achieve the desired expansion of the vascular compartment (as only one-quarter to one-third remains). However, while they may be relatively inefficient, isotonic crystalloids have been shown to be effective in achieving resuscitation (Cazzolli and Prittie, 2015). Further, the interstitial shift of fluids may be beneficial for patients that are concurrently dehydrated. The biggest drawback to isotonic crystalloids is the potential to promote tissue edema and create acid–base disturbances with large-volume administration.

Within isotonic crystalloids there are the balanced electrolyte solutions (e.g., Plasma-Lyte and lactate Ringer's solution) and "physiological saline" (0.9% NaCl). For decades they were thought to be interchangeable, but more recent evidence suggests that the potential for hyperchloremic metabolic acidosis caused by 0.9% NaCl may be associated with an increased risk of acute kidney injury (Semler and Kellum, 2019). As such, unless the patient has significant hypochloremia, use of a balanced electrolyte solution is recommended over 0.9% NaCl.

6i.2.3 Hypertonic crystalloids

Hypertonic crystalloids (e.g., 7% NaCl) are hyperosmolar compared with the patient. The potential benefit of these fluids is that they promote a shift of fluid into the vascular compartment, thereby resulting in a volume expansion much larger than the amount given. Historically this is reported to be anywhere from 4 to 6 times, though a study in dogs showed the overall expansion to be much less (Silverstein *et al.*, 2005). However, a recent study in cats did demonstrate that 5% hypertonic saline (HTS) was 6 times more potent at achieving volume expansion compared with an isotonic crystalloid (Yiew *et al.*, 2020). In either circumstance, the volume of HTS administered will redistribute across the extracellular space within the space of 30–60 min. As a result, the effect of HTS will be short-lived and will not result in a sustained volume expansion. With this in mind, HTS is best served in circumstances of impending cardiovascular collapse to "buy time" while other fluids are administered. Patients with traumatic brain injury, particularly in conjunction with hypotension, may also benefit from the dual effect of HTS to expand vascular volume and promote osmotic reduction in intracranial pressure.

Table 6i.3. Recommended uses for various fluid types in resuscitation.

Fluid type	Recommended use
Hypotonic crystalloid	Contraindicated
Balanced electrolyte solution	General-purpose resuscitation fluid, especially with dehydration
0.9 % NaCl	Hypochloremic metabolic alkalosis, otherwise not recommended
Hypertonic saline	Impending cardiovascular collapse Traumatic brain injury
Synthetic colloid	Not recommended unless natural colloids unavailable
Natural colloid, blood products	Hypoproteinemia Hemorrhage

6i.2.4 Synthetic or natural colloids

Colloid solutions typically contain macromolecules (>10 kDA) suspended in crystalloid solution. As such they contribute to oncotic pressure and are theoretically more likely to remain within the vascular compartment and exert a more sustained effect compared with crystalloids (see Chapter 4). For this reason, it has been suggested that each 1 ml of colloid administered will result in an increase of 1–1.5 ml of circulating volume. This would make them seem ideally suited to the primary goal of fluid resuscitation—expansion of the vascular volume—especially in patients experiencing blood loss and/or hypoproteinemia. Despite this, a clear benefit of colloid administration over crystalloids has not been demonstrated in human or veterinary medicine (Cazzolli and Prittie, 2015; Adamik and Yozova, 2021). This may be at least partly because colloids do not remain within the vascular space to quite the extent that was previously believed. As described in Chapter 2, the classic notion of Starling's forces (hydrostatic and oncotic pressure, vascular permeability) has undergone significant revision. The endothelial surface layer (ESL), comprising the endothelium and the glycocalyx, provides the true "barrier", with hydrostatic pressure being the primary determinant and lymphatic drainage maintaining the balance. However, with any disruption of the ESL (such as with inflammatory disease or aggressive fluid administration), colloids can more readily move into the interstitium. This means a less effective increase in circulating volume and the potential to worsen interstitial edema.

Within the category of colloids, there is also consideration of synthetic (e.g., VetStarch) versus natural (e.g., albumin or plasma products). Synthetic colloids carry the benefit of long shelf-life without need for specific storage or access to blood donors or blood products. However, significant concerns have been raised regarding the potential for synthetic colloids to cause and/or contribute to coagulopathy and acute kidney injury. While most of the evidence for the latter has come from human medicine, the potential risk has also resulted in significant reduction to almost complete cessation of their use in veterinary medicine (Cazzolli and Prittie, 2015; Adamik and Yozova, 2021). That said, for patients not responding to crystalloids, use of synthetic colloids may be considered, especially when natural colloids are not available (Adamik and Yozova, 2021). Ongoing administration of synthetic colloids for oncotic support is not recommended.

In this regard the use of natural colloids has increased significantly, both for acute resuscitation and for ongoing oncotic support (Culler *et al.*, 2019; Adamik and Yozova, 2021). This can include canine or human albumin products, or plasma-based products (fresh frozen plasma, frozen plasma, cryo-poor plasma, fresh whole blood). See Chapter 4ii for more information on each of these products. Briefly, 10% canine albumin products are in limited supply but offer the benefit of being species-specific and thereby carry a lower risk of immune reaction. Human albumin is more readily available but is only 80% similar to canine albumin. As such, both acute and delayed hypersensitivity have been reported in dogs administered human albumin. While this is especially true in healthy dogs, it has also been reported in critically ill patients (Adamik and Yozova, 2021). In addition, the hyperoncotic nature of 25% human albumin could be associated with volume overload if given rapidly. Plasma products can carry the benefit of volume expansion and albumin supplementation, as well as the ability to replenish coagulation factors. Limitations are availability, cost, and the potential for transfusion reactions.

6i.2.5 Red blood cell transfusion

Specific to hemorrhagic or anemic shock, administration of red blood cells (either fresh whole blood or packed red blood cells) may be necessary as part of resuscitation fluid therapy. This would especially be the case for bleeding patients not responding to an initial dose of crystalloids or colloids, or those experiencing catastrophic hemorrhage and needing massive transfusion. Full consideration of transfusion medicine and delivery of these products is beyond the scope of this chapter, but is covered in more detail in Chapter 8i, as well as in other resources (Linklater, 2019; Hall and Drobatz, 2021)

6i.3 Routes of Administration for Resuscitation

Given the nature and goal of fluid resuscitation, the route of delivery needs to allow for rapid administration of relatively large volumes. In this regard, intravenous access will be needed, and the subcutaneous and enteral routes will not be effective (see Chapter 5 for more information). In order to optimize flow, ideally the largest bore and shortest catheter should be utilized. In addition, cephalic or jugular catheter placement is preferred, as this puts the point of administration closer to the heart/central circulation. Further, this helps to make it less likely that the fluids could be trapped behind a process obstructing venous return (such as gastric dilatation and volvulus). For very large patients, it may be necessary to place two catheters for simultaneous delivery to achieve the volume needed in the desired period of time. If intravenous access cannot be achieved, it may be necessary to consider intraosseous (IO) catheter placement or performing a vascular cut-down procedure. It is important to note that these are equivalent forms of access: anything that can be given IV can be given IO. See Box 6i.2 for a summary of these ideal characteristics for resuscitation fluid administration.

In addition to gaining vascular access, there can also be logistical considerations with regard to the volume of fluid that needs to be given over the desired time. Ideally a volumetric pump is used to help ensure more accurate delivery. However, most pumps have a maximum rate of 999 ml/h. If a faster rate is needed, administration could potentially be spread over two pumps delivered through two catheters (for a total rate of about 2 l/h). Another consideration is the use of a pressure bag (or "slam" bag) around the fluids with straight infusion into the patient (Fig. 6i.3). This system can potentially deliver 1 l of fluids in under 7 min. However, the general trend and recommendation in fluid resuscitation is toward lower volumes and slower rates of administration (as will be discussed below). As such, it is uncommonly necessary to deliver fluids that quickly except in extreme circumstances.

Box 6i.2. Ideal characteristics for delivery of fluid resuscitation.

- Intravenous
  - Cephalic or jugular preferred over saphenous
  - Large bore, short length
  - Two catheters may be needed for large/giant breed dogs
- Intraosseous as an alternative if venous access not possible

6i.4 How Much/How Fast? Classic Approach

The classic approach to fluid resuscitation is largely based on the notion that restoring circulating volume as quickly as possible is ideal. The associated volumes and rates of delivery are based on the circulating **blood volume** (about 80 ml/kg for dogs, about 50 ml/kg for cats), the **presumed loss** (expected to be at least 30% to demonstrate signs of shock), and the relative **"efficiency"** of the fluid (the increase in circulating volume for each milliliter administered). These factors combine to give the **"total shock dose"**, or the total amount that might need to be given in order to achieve the desired volume expansion. Here is an example of how these are calculated using dogs and isotonic crystalloids:

V = 80 ml/kg (blood volume) × 0.3 (presumed loss) / 1/3–1/4 (efficiency)

V = ~70–90 ml/kg

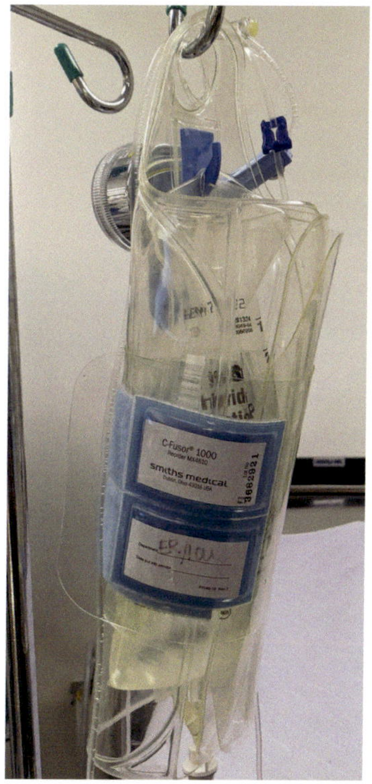

Fig. 6i.3. Pressure bag used to facilitate rapid delivery of intravenous fluids.

Based on this, the total shock dose winds up being close to the circulating blood volume. Again, this is meant to reflect the relative inefficiency of isotonic crystalloids, not that a full blood volume has been lost. In addition, there will have been some loss from the interstitium as fluid shifts in response to hypovolemia. These calculations can be performed for each fluid type to determine the total shock dose for each of the other fluid types (Table 6i.4). It is important to recognize that these values are meant to serve as rough guidelines, and that the actual volume needed may vary considerably based on the individual patient and underlying disease process. To this end, the total shock dose is titrated to effect, giving some fraction of the total shock dose over some period time and reassessing. Classically this meant that clinicians would bolus one-quarter to one-third of the shock dose over 15–20 min for isotonic crystalloids and colloids (Table 6i.4). The bolus would be repeated until the resuscitation goals were met, or a total shock dose was given. If the patient had still not responded, then it might be necessary to try a different type of fluid (such as blood products), or try other interventions (such as pressors, inotropes, etc.). This approach was supported by early experimental hemorrhage which suggested that it was necessary to administer three times the amount of blood lost in order to achieve resuscitation (the **3-to-1 rule**) (Santry and Alam, 2010). In addition, the widely accepted early goal-directed therapy (EGDT) bundle for sepsis included a starting bolus of 30 ml/kg for patients in septic shock (Rivers *et al.*, 2001).

The approach to administration of HTS is different from that for isotonic crystalloids and colloids. Given that the goal of HTS is acute volume expansion through osmotic pull, it has to be given more quickly (over 5–10 min), otherwise it will start to redistribute and lose the effect. However, HTS should not be given any faster than this timeframe (0.5–1 ml/kg/min) because of the concern that acute volume expansion can trigger a reflex bradycardia. It is also important to note that the dosing of HTS is based on using a 7–7.5% solution. As it often comes stocked as a 23.4% solution in small animal clinical settings, this *must* be diluted to the target range. This can be accomplished by diluting the stock solution approximately 1:2 with sterile water or isotonic crystalloid. A synthetic colloid could also be used to dilute the 23.4% hypertonic saline to create a combination hypertonic/oncotic resuscitation fluid (so-called "turbostarch"). The potential benefit would be the acute volume expansion of the HTS with the more sustained effect of the synthetic colloid. It is dosed the same as HTS and given over the same time frame.

6i.5 How Much/How Fast? Revised Approach

The classic approach previously described has been used for decades with the goal of achieving rapid restoration of circulating volume and resolution of shock. However, more recently this approach has been called into question with the concern that large-volume rapid administration of fluids (particularly isotonic crystalloids) may have some adverse effects. This notion first came to the forefront in circumstances of the actively bleeding patient. While initially it seems intuitive that the bleeding patient needs volume replaced rapidly, doing so with non-blood products (crystalloids,

Table 6i.4. Classic and revised doses for fluid resuscitation

Fluid	Efficiency	Classic total shock dose (ml/kg)			Initial bolus (ml/kg)	
					Classic	Revised
Isotonic crystalloid	0.25–0.33	Dog	70–90	Dog	20–30	10–15
		Cat	40–60	Cat	10–15	5–10
HTS (7–7.5%) ("turbostarch")	4–6	Dog	3–6	Dog	3–6	N/A
		Cat	2–4	Cat	2–4	N/A
Colloid (synthetic or plasma)	1–1.5	Dog	15–25	Dog	5	2–3
		Cat	10–15	Cat	3–4	1–2

Efficiency reflects the increase in vascular volume for each milliliter administered. Bolus given over 15–20 min in the classic approach, 20–30 min in the revised approach for isotonic crystalloids and colloids. Hypertonic saline (HTS) given over 5–10 min. "Turbostarch" is the 1:2 combination of 23.4% HTS and synthetic colloid.

synthetic colloids) can result in hemodilution, worsening coagulopathy, and exacerbation of hemorrhage (Dutton, 2007). The latter is attributed to increased perfusion pressure and dislodging clots (see Chapter 8i for more information on fluid therapy in hemorrhage/trauma). In these circumstances the potential benefits of a more cautious approach to fluid therapy start to make sense, but it is less clear how this applies to other circumstances of fluid resuscitation (such as sepsis, obstructive shock, severe dehydration). To answer this, it becomes important to consider some of the other impacts that large-volume rapid administration of fluids can have.

In Chapter 2 there is discussion of Starling's forces in the context of the balance of fluid between the intravascular and interstitial spaces. Based on these concepts, acute administration of isotonic crystalloid should result in an increase in hydrostatic pressure and decrease in oncotic pressure (through dilution). In addition, rapid administration of large volumes of fluid may cause shedding of the glycocalyx from the endothelial surface layer (Smart and Hughes, 2021). This is believed to be secondary to shearing force, hemodilution, and an increase in natriuretic peptide release triggered by acute volume expansion (Smart and Hughes, 2021). When combined with the potential for inflammation and shock to also negatively impact the glycocalyx, the stage is set for a significant disruption of the endothelial surface layer. The resulting increase in permeability, along with an increase in hydrostatic pressure and decrease in oncotic pressure, can then result in more dramatic loss of fluid to the interstitial space. This can be reflected by the development of significant tissue edema and resultant disruption of organ function (Cotton *et al.*, 2006). Taking all this into account, it may be reasonable to consider a less-is-more approach to fluid resuscitation. There is evidence from human medicine to support a more restrictive approach to fluid resuscitation, particularly in hemorrhagic and septic shock, though there are conflicting results (Self *et al.*, 2018; Jiang *et al.*, 2021). To date there have not been any clinical studies looking at large-volume resuscitation compared with a more conservative fluid administration in veterinary patients.

So, what does a "revised" approach look like? The key difference is the volume given (less) and the time-frame of administration (slower). As no specific guidelines have been established, a reasonable starting point for "less" is half the dose given in the classic approach (e.g., an isotonic crystalloid at 10–15 ml/kg rather than 20–30 ml/kg) administered over a similar or "slower" period of time (e.g., 20–30 min instead of 15–20 min). The end result is a "**slowless**" rather than a bolus. As in the classic approach, fluids are still carefully titrated to achieve the goals of resuscitation: stabilization and improvement of the clinical signs and other markers associated with shock (see below). The slowless can be given 2–3 times before deciding whether additional fluid administration is likely to be helpful, or if other interventions are needed (such as pressors, inotropes, blood products, etc). With this approach it is much less likely that the classic total shock dose (or even half of that) will be reached. While prospective studies are still needed, clinical experience with this approach has yielded success in achieving resuscitation with significantly less fluid administration. Figure 6i.4 provides a suggested algorithm.

An exception to the application of this revised approach is the patient that is experiencing impending cardiovascular collapse (e.g., terminal shock, catastrophic hemorrhage). In these circumstances (late decompensated to terminal shock) there might not be sufficient time for a slowless, and the classic approach might be needed. Another key aspect of this revised approach is earlier consideration of blood products in the bleeding patient, or earlier use of pressors in patients with maldistributive (septic) shock. See Chapters 8i and 8ii for more information.

6i.6 Monitoring and Resuscitation Endpoints

Regardless of which approach is taken, frequent monitoring is essential for careful titration of fluids and to achieve the endpoints of resuscitation. Many of the parameters that need to be assessed have already been discussed in the context of shock recognition (Table 6i.2 and Box 6i.1). While improvement in blood pressure is an important step in the right direction, it does not necessarily signal the end of resuscitation. As previously discussed, blood pressure is the last thing to go, and so it is the first thing to come back. Fixing the blood pressure does not mean that shock has been resolved, but more that the patient has moved from decompensated to compensated. Continued assessment with the goal of improving the perfusion parameters like heart rate, mucous membrane

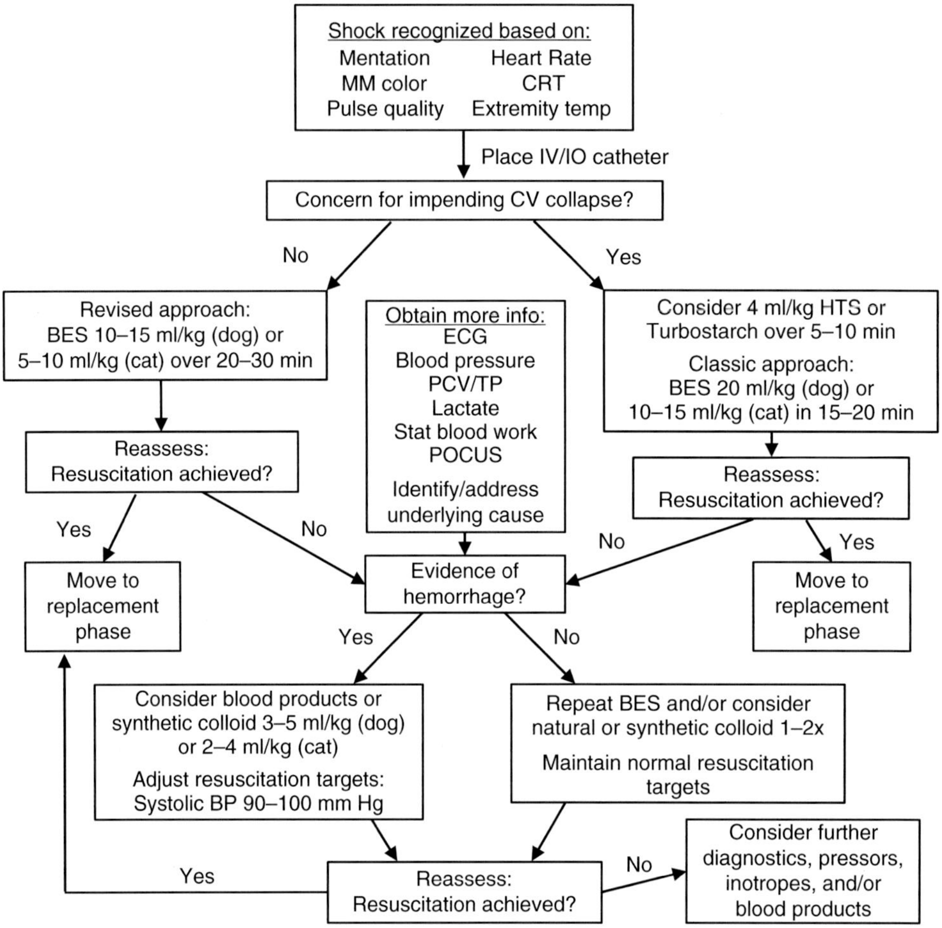

Fig. 6i.4. Algorithm with suggested approach to fluid resuscitation. BES, balanced electrolyte solution; CRT, capillary refill time; CV, cardiovascular; HTS, hypertonic saline; IO, intraosseous; IV, intravenous; MM, mucous membranes; PCV/TP, packed cell volume/total protein; POCUS, point-of-care ultrasound. Note: Impending cardiovascular collapse signifies late decompensated to terminal shock.

color, capillary refill time, and peripheral pulse quality is essential also to ensure that resuscitation has been achieved. In this regard continuous ECG can be very helpful to visually assess the impact of fluid therapy on a moment-to-moment basis. Combining heart rate and blood pressure to determine shock index (HR/SBP) and track over time can also be an effective way to gauge response (ideally seeing it drop below 1.0).

Serial measurement of lactate to determine clearance can be very helpful in guiding fluid therapy and gauging severity. It may also help to reflect occult hypoperfusion or ischemia that is not evident based on heart rate or blood pressure. Based on its half-life, it can be expected that hyperlactatemia should decrease by 50% every 1–2 h and resolve within 6–12 h (Rosenstein *et al.*, 2018). Monitoring central venous saturation (SvO_2) has also been utilized as a marker of tissue oxygen balance, with the notion that increased oxygen extraction (lower SvO_2) suggests a greater oxygen debt. This was one of the cornerstones of EGDT in septic patients, with a target of >70% (Rivers *et al.*, 2001). However, subsequent studies have failed to replicate the survival benefit of EGDT. Obtaining SvO_2 also requires placement of a central venous catheter (as the sample needs to come from the vena cava, not a peripheral vessel) and a blood-gas analyzer, both of which may be unavailable and/or impractical in many veterinary clinics. Comparably, the ability to measure lactate with a hand-held lactometer is typically much more feasible. With these limitations, it is unclear what role monitoring SvO_2 might play as a resuscitation endpoint in veterinary medicine. Repeated monitoring of PCV/TP can offer insight regarding progress toward resolution of hemoconcentration from severe dehydration, or trigger a potential need for blood products/oncotic support with progressive anemia/hypoproteinemia.

A notable exception to the goal of normalizing these endpoints as quickly as possible is the patient with active hemorrhage. As alluded to previously, there is potential to exacerbate bleeding with aggressive resuscitative efforts and even just trying to achieve a normal blood pressure. In this regard the notion of a more restrictive or hypotensive resuscitation has been put forth for patients in hemorrhagic shock. In this approach the goals are set lower by targeting a minimally acceptable (i.e., systolic pressure of 80–100 mm Hg) rather than a normal blood pressure. The other parameters (heart rate, mucous membranes, etc.) are allowed to be abnormal until hemostasis is achieved. See Chapter 8i for more information.

6i.7 Conclusion

Fluid resuscitation plays a major role in treating the most common causes of shock (e.g. hypovolemia). Early recognition of shock is essential for timely initiation of fluid therapy in order to limit the negative impacts of shock while seeking to determine the underlying cause. An isotonic crystalloid is a reasonable starting point for most circumstances given that these are readily available, low-cost, and reasonably effective. A revised, less-is-more approach to volume and rate of administration is recommended, with the notion that it may be more effective unless there is concern for impending cardiovascular collapse. Once resuscitation has been initiated, frequent monitoring and reassessment are needed to gauge response and determine if additional volume and/or other fluid types may be needed. If target endpoints have been reached, the resuscitation phase of fluid therapy can be stopped with transition to the replacement or maintenance phase. If two to three rounds of slowless/bolus do not result in effective resuscitation, it may be necessary to consider other interventions based on the suspected or confirmed underlying cause (e.g., blood products, pressors, inotropes, etc.). This general approach to fluid resuscitation is presented in Fig. 6i.4.

Clinical Case 6i.1

A 9-month-old FS mixed-breed dog (weighing 10 kg) presents for 2–3 days of vomiting and bloody diarrhea. Based on signalment and vaccination status there is a strong suspicion for parvoviral enteritis. Her initial vitals are as follows:

HR 170, RR 48, Temp 103.2
Pulse quality decreased, MM pale pink, CRT 3 sec
8% dehydration
Mentation QAR
Doppler blood pressure – 110 mm Hg

Though her blood pressure is normal, you recognize that she has abnormal perfusion parameters, and so determine that she is likely in compensated hypovolemic shock secondary to dehydration. As a result, resuscitation fluid therapy is indicated, so an intravenous catheter is placed. Given her dehydration from GI losses, you choose a balanced electrolyte solution (Plasma-Lyte) to start your resuscitation using the revised approach:

Revised isotonic crystalloid = 10–15 ml/kg × 10 kg
= 100–150 ml given over 20–30 min

Since she is still normotensive, you decide to go lower and slower and give 100 ml over 30 min, using a volumetric pump (rate 200 ml/h with volume to be infused of 100 ml). As the slowless finishes, you reassess her vitals:

HR 130, RR 36, Temp 102.8
Pulse quality moderate, MM pink, CRT 2 sec
8% dehydration
Mentation QAR
Doppler blood pressure – 130 mm Hg

In addition to her blood pressure, her perfusion parameters have improved, and she is no longer in shock. Further resuscitation is not needed, and she can transition to the replacement phase of fluid therapy.

Clinical Case 6i.2

A 6-year-old MC Maltese (weighing 3 kg) presents for an acute onset of vomiting and collapse. The owners live an hour away, and he started having bloody "raspberry jam" diarrhea and becoming progressively less responsive on the way. Here are his initial vitals:

HR 50, RR 24, Temp 95.0
PQ unable to feel, MM pale/white, CRT > 4 sec
10–12% dehydration
Mentation stuporous

Based on these findings, you are concerned that he is in late decompensated to terminal hypovolemic shock. Given the impending cardiovascular collapse, an IV catheter is placed, and you decide to administer "turbostarch" for rapid volume expansion, as well as a "classic" bolus of isotonic crystalloids:

Turbostarch dose = 3–6 ml/kg. Decide to give 4 ml/kg × 3 kg = 12 ml given over 5 min

To create turbostarch, dilute 4 ml of the 23.4% HTS stock solution with 8 ml VetStarch (1:2 dilution).

Classic isotonic crystalloid = 20–30 ml/kg × 3 kg = 60–90 ml given over 15–20 min.

Since turbostarch is also being given, you decide to give 60 ml over 20 min using a volumetric pump (rate 180 ml/h with volume to be infused of 60 ml).

Once the bolus of isotonic crystalloids is finished you reassess vitals and additional information has been obtained:

HR 160, RR 40, Temp 99.0
PQ weak, MM pale pink, CRT 3–4 sec
10% dehydration
Mentation dull
Doppler blood pressure – 60mm Hg
PCV/TP (from catheter, before fluids) – 71%/5.0 g/dl
Lactate 8.3 mmol/l

The patient has shown improvement but is still in decompensated shock. Given the clinical signs and PCV/TP you are concerned about acute hemorrhagic diarrhea syndrome, with rapid loss of protein-rich fluid from vascular volume into the GI tract. As the total protein has likely dropped further with fluid administration, it is decided to use a natural colloid (fresh frozen plasma) for the next round of fluid resuscitation. The patient is still fairly decompensated, so you decide to go with a "classic" dose:

Classic colloid = 5 ml/kg × 3 kg = 15 ml plasma given over 20 min.

The patient's cardiovascular status improves (Doppler 100 mm Hg), but he is still showing signs of shock (tachycardia, pale pink mucous membranes, CRT 2–3 sec). Recheck PCV/TP 62%/4.2 g/dl, lactate 3.9 mmol/l. It is decided to give another dose of plasma, but as the patient is more stable the "revised" approach is taken:

Revised colloid = 3 ml/kg × 3 kg = 9 ml plasma given over 30 min.

Afterward Doppler 110, the patient's heart rate, mucous membranes, and CRT have improved. You decide that he does not need any further resuscitation and move into the replacement phase of fluid therapy.

See Chapter 8i for a case example of fluid resuscitation in hemorrhagic shock, and Chapter 8ii for a case example of fluid resuscitation in septic shock.

References

Adamik, K.-N. and Yozova, E.D. (2021) Colloids yes or no? – a "Gretchen question" answered. *Frontiers in Veterinary Science* 8, 624049.

Cazzolli, D. and Prittie, J. (2015) The crystalloid-colloid debate: consequences of resuscitation fluid slelection in veterinary critical care. *Journal of Veterinary Emergency and Critical Care* 25(1), 6–19.

Cooper, E.S. (2019) Pathophysiology of shock. In: Drobatz, K.J., Hopper, K., Rozanski, E. and Silverstein, D.C. (eds) *Textbook of Small Animal Emergency Medicine*. John Wiley and Sons, Hoboken, New Jersey, pp. 981–985.

Cotton, B.A., Guy, J.S., Morris, J.A. *et al.* (2006) The cellular, metabolic, and systemic consequences of aggressive fluid resuscitation strategies. *Shock* 26(2), 115–121.

Culler, C.A., Balakrishnan, A., Yaxley, P.E. and Guiallumin, J. (2019) Clinical use of cyropoor plasma continuous rate infusion in critically ill, hypoabluminemic dogs. *Journal of Veterinary Emergency and Critical Care* 29(3), 314–320.

Dutton, R.P. (2007) Current concepts in hemorrhagic shock. *Anesthesiology Clinics* 25, 23–34.

Hall, K. and Drobatz, K. (2021) Volume resuscitation in the acute hemorrhaging patient: historic use to current applications. *Frontiers in Veterinary Science* 8, 638104.

Jiang, S., Wu, M., Lu, X. *et al.* (2021) Is restrictive fluid resuscitation beneficial not only for hemorrhagic shock but also for septic shock? A meta-analysis. *Medicine (Baltimore)* 100(12), e25143.

Linklater, A. (2019) Management of hemorrhagic shock. In: Drobatz, K.J., Hopper, K., Rozanski, E. and Silverstein, D.C. (eds) *Textbook of Small Animal Emergency Medicine.* John Wiley and Sons, Hoboken, New Jersey, pp. 1115–1125.

Lisciandro, G.R. and Lisciandro, S.C. (2021) Global FAST for patient monitoring and staging in dogs and cats. *Veterinary Clinics of North America Small Animal Practice* 51(6), 1315–1333.

Muir, W.W. (2006) Trauma: physiology, pathophysiology, and clinical implications. *Journal of Veterinary Emergency and Critical Care* 16(4), 253–263.

Peterson, K.L., Hardy, B.T. and Hall, K. (2013) Assessment of shock index in healthy dogs and dogs in hemorrhagic shock. *Journal of Veterinary Emergency and Critical Care* 23, 545–550.

Porter, A.E., Rozanski, E.A., Sharp, C.R. *et al.* (2013) Evaluation of the shock index in dogs presenting as emergencies. *Journal of Veterinary Emergency and Critical Care* 23, 538–544.

Rivers, E., Nguyen, B., Havstad, S. *et al.* (2001) Early goal-directed therapy in the treatment of severe sepsis and septic shock. *New England Journal of Medicine* 345, 1368–1377.

Rosenstein, P.G., Tennet-Brown, B.S. and Hughes, D. (2018) Clinical use of plasma lactate concentration. Part 2: Prognostic and diagnostic utility and the clinical management of hyperlactatemia. *Journal of Veterinary Emergency and Critical Care* 28(2), 106–121.

Santry, H.P. and Alam, H.B. (2010) Fluid resuscitation: past, present, and the future. *Shock* 33(3), 229–241.

Self, W.H., Semler, M.W., Bellomo, R. *et al.* (2018) Liberal versus restrictive intravenous fluid therapy for early septic shock: rationale for a randomized trial. *Annals of Emergency Medicine* 72(4), 457–466.

Semler, M.W. and Kellum, J.A. (2019) Balanced crystalloid solutions. *American Journal of Respiratory and Critical Care Medicine* 199(8), 952–960.

Silverstein, D.C., Aldrich, J., Haskins, S.C. *et al.* (2005) Assessment of changes in blood volume in response to resuscitative fluid administration in dogs. *Journal of Veterinary Emergency and Critical Care* 15, 185–192.

Smart, L. and Hughes, D. (2021) The effects of resuscitative fluid therapy on the endothelial surface layer. *Frontiers in Veterinary Science* 8, 661660.

Waddell, L.S. and Brown, A.J. (2015) Hemodynamic monitoring. In: Silverstein, D.C. and Hopper, K. (eds) *Small Animal Critical Care Medicine*, 2nd edn. Elsevier, Philadelphia, Pennsylvania, pp. 51–54.

Williamson, J.A. and Leone, S. (2012) Noninvasive arterial blood pressure monitoring. In: Burkitt Creedon, J.M. and Davis, H. (eds) *Advanced Monitoring and Procedures for Small Animal Emergency and Critical Care*. Wiley and Sons, Hoboken, New Jersey, pp. 134–144.

Yiew, X.T., Bateman, S.W., Hahn, R.G. and Bersenas, A.M.E. (2020) Evaluation of the distribution and elimination of balanced isotonic crystalloid, 5% hypertonic saline, and 6% tetrastarch 130/0.4 using volume kinetic modeling and analysis in healthy conscious cats. *Frontiers in Veterinary Science* 7, 587564.

6ii Replacement Fluid Therapy

Julien Guillaumin

Colorado State University, Fort Collins, Colorado, USA

The replacement phase of fluid therapy is geared toward returning any fluid deficits the patient has experienced by the time of presentation (**dehydration**), as well as keeping up with any continued loss of fluid from the body (**ongoing losses**), and providing for daily fluid needs (**maintenance**). This phase would typically be enacted after resuscitation had been completed, or if resuscitation was not needed and there was clinical concern for dehydration and the presence of ongoing losses. In order to determine how to calculate replacement fluid rates, assessment of dehydration and approaches to quantifying ongoing losses must be considered.

6ii.1 Dehydration

There are multiple ways to define dehydration. In its narrower sense, coined in 1800 by the French chemist Joseph-Louis Proust (1754–1826), and its Greek etymology, dehydration can be defined by a lack of free water, or hypotonic fluid loss.

However, when clinicians assess and treat dehydration, they are assessing interstitial tissues, part of the extracellular fluid space, and replace dehydration with isotonic fluids. Therefore, for the purpose of clinical practice, dehydration should be defined as a loss of isotonic fluid (i.e., salt and water), or extracellular fluid compartment (DiBartola and Bateman, 2006). The purist should use the term “extracellular fluid dehydration”, as opposed to “intracellular fluid dehydration”, which is the loss of free water, and is characterized by hypernatremia, with minimal evidence of “clinical” dehydration.

6ii.1.1 General assessment of dehydration

Estimating dehydration from physical examination is very crude and is extrapolated from historical experiments in dogs. In those experiments, healthy dogs were given furosemide, which generates isotonic fluid loss, and serial physical examinations were done. For example, a 10 kg healthy Beagle which would lose 0.5 kg (or 5% of its body weight) would have physical examination findings consistent with 5% dehydration. Those early experiments generated tables such as Table 6ii.1, which are still in use today (Wellman *et al.*, 2006).

In general, most clinicians believe that physical examination using the classic signs of mucous membrane moistness, skin elasticity, and eye position in the orbit would provide an estimate within 5% of the dehydrated. For example, if you believe based on your physical examination that the patient is 5% dehydrated, it may range from not dehydrated at all (i.e., 0%) to more severely dehydrated (i.e., 10%). Most clinicians also believe that you cannot detect less than 5% dehydration. So, if the 10 kg healthy Beagle has lost 3% of its body weight due to dehydration, its physical examination would be mostly normal. Therefore, it is recommended that clinicians use several parameters to assess dehydration, not just one aspect, and recognize the limitations of each.

The **history** can give some clues about the hydration status of the patient. Patients presented with known gastrointestinal losses (e.g., vomiting, diarrhea, hypersalivating), respiratory losses (e.g., panting), and urinary losses (e.g., excessive urination, especially without compensation by drinking) are probably dehydrated. Patients with severe burns, no access to water and in warm and/or dry weather may also point the clinician towards a suspicion of dehydration. Excessive insensible water losses (e.g., panting, fever), or third-space losses (e.g., ascites, pleural effusion) can be determined from history and physical examination findings. The time period over which fluid losses have occurred should also be determined, as it plays a role in replacing the lost fluid.

Physical examination findings are commonly used to assess dehydration. It can be important to realize that none of these physical examination findings will give 100% sensitivity or specificity for

DOI: 10.1079/9781789243406.0062

Table 6ii.1. Estimation of dehydration based on physical examination findings, and its correlation with changes in body weight.

Estimated dehydration	Changes in body weight	Thirst present	Mucous membrane	Skin elasticity	Eye in orbit	Signs of hypovolemia
Mild	5–7%	Yes	Tacky	Slightly decrease	Normal position	No
Moderate	8–10%	Yes	Tacky	Decrease	May be sunken	No
Severe	10–12%	Yes	Tacky	Stands in a fold	Sunken eyes	Yes

the dehydration of the patient. As mentioned above, our clinical ability to assess dehydration is poor. The clinician should go through multiple steps in order to generate and monitor fluid therapy plans, as follows.

- Integrate patient history and physical examination findings.
- Commit to a certain dehydration level.
- Generate the fluid therapy planning and implement it.
- Monitor the patient carefully until rehydration is evident.

6ii.1.2 Physical examination findings of dehydration

We can use six **hydration parameters** based on physical examination findings and behavior modifications in order to assess dehydration (Table 6ii.1). The clinician can estimate the hydration deficit by evaluation of the mucous membrane moistness, the skin elasticity (where decreased elasticity, or turgidity, is related to increased time for a skin tent to return to normal position), the position of the eye in the orbit, changes in body weight, as well as intravascular volume status. Decreased intravascular volume, or shock, can be identified by perfusion parameters such as heart rate, capillary refill time, mucous membrane color, pulse quality, extremity temperature and level of consciousness (see Chapter 6i). Presence of a thirst mechanism completes the assessment of the hydration status. Clinicians then use tables to "commit" to a certain dehydration plan (Table 6ii.1).

No single "hydration parameter" is only influenced by hydration status. A review of each individual hydration parameter with emphasis on limitations is helpful in making these assessments, as follows.

Mucous membrane moistness

The amount of saliva and tear film varies inversely with hydration status. It is a qualitative measurement: moistness of finger or glove, "shiny" mucous membranes, lachrymal lake, etc. It is influenced by evaporation (e.g., panting; fan in front of the dog; dry climate), other disease processes such as oral ulceration due to trauma, infection or uremia, and tear production influenced by other local factors such as keratoconjunctivitis sicca.

Skin elasticity test

The skin's elasticity depends on hydration status. The return to the normal position when a skin fold is pulled from the thorax depends on the interstitial fluid component. That is why we define hydration as a loss of extracellular fluid volume for the purpose of clinical assessment of dehydration. If it is slow to return, there is lack or elasticity (i.e., turgor) and the animal is dehydrated. It also can assess overhydration, if the interstitial fluid is very jelly-like. Aside from hydration status, skin elasticity is influenced by age, with youth having increased skin elasticity compared with geriatric patients, as well as body fat, with obese patient having an increased interstitial fluid volume and skin elasticity. Breed can also influence a patient's skin elasticity, as skin thickness influences the time for the skin fold to return to a normal position.

Eye position in orbit

The position of the eyeball can correspond to loss of periorbital/retro-orbital fat and is directly correlated with hydration status (Fig. 6ii.1). It can be influenced by ocular disease (e.g., microphthalmia, buphthalmos, exophthalmos) and body condition score, or nutritional status of the patient. It is a late finding in dehydrated animals.

Changes in body weight

Our entire current assessment of hydration is based on earlier canine studies on normal research

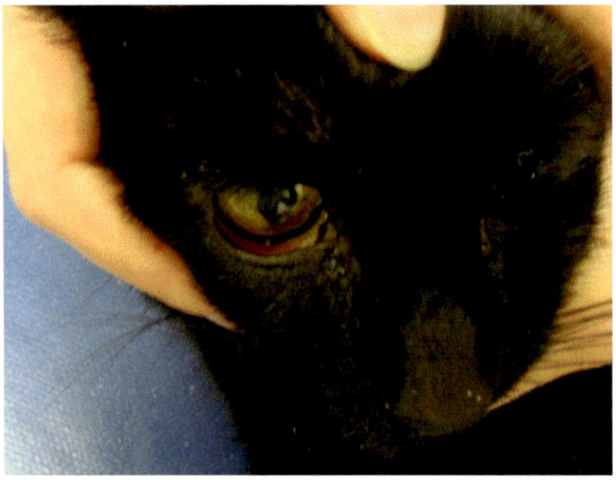

Fig. 6ii.1. Position of the eye in the orbit is one of the parameters that can be used for assessment of dehydration. Extracellular fluid dehydration reduces the size of the orbital fat pad and the eyeball sinks into the orbit.

dogs: normal dogs were used, with no access to food and water. Dehydration was induced by use of diuretics and body weight was monitored and compared with physical examination findings. Body weight changes are also obviously influenced by change in lean body mass. However, weight changes over a short period of time (i.e., hours or over the space of a day) are more likely to reflect changes in body water. Although body weight is the most accurate of the physical examination findings, it is rarely practical for assessment of dehydration, as it is unusual for the clinician to have the patient's current and exact body weight *before* being dehydrated. However, a body weight change is one of the best ways the clinician can assess and monitor rehydration status: corrected 5% dehydration should increase the patient's body weight by 5%.

Example:

If a patient weighs 20 kg and is believed to be 5% dehydrated, the expected deficit is 1 l (20 × 0.05 = 1 l). So the fully rehydrated patient should then weigh 21 kg, having gained 1 l (1 kg) of fluid.

Thirst

Thirst is a sensation that is difficult to describe, and even more difficult to detect in dogs and cats. However, the thirst centers are triggered by two mechanisms. The first one is a **decrease in the extracellular fluid volume**, which we defined as dehydration: the baroreceptors in the aortic arch and carotid sinus sense a decrease in volume and signal the brain to initiate the search for water and to increase the release of ADH. It also triggers the renin–angiotensin–aldosterone system (RAAS). Angiotensin II is vasoactive and triggers aldosterone release, but also stimulates the thirst centers in the brain to search out and ingest water. Aldosterone is the hormone of sodium regulation and acts on the kidneys (reabsorption of salt and water) and the brain (sensitizing it to the action of angiotension II).

The second mechanism is an **increase in osmolality of the extracellular space** (i.e., an increase in the concentration of sodium) which, sensed by the osmoreceptors, initiates the act of searching for water (or a food with a large percentage of water) and then the behavioral act of drinking. However, in these circumstances patients are expected to be hypernatremic and are lacking intracellular fluid volume, and usually show minimal clinical signs of extracellular fluid deficit. Hypernatremic patients should receive free water to correct their intracellular fluid volume deficit (see Chapter 8vi).

Signs of hypovolemia

So far, we have assumed that dehydration was equivalent to the loss from the isotonic fluid compartment, and we have used our physical examination skills to "interrogate" the interstitial fluid compartment. Although most of our physical examination findings are related to the interstitial fluid compartment, with dehydration the fluid is lost from the entire extracellular space, including the intravenous fluid compartment. However, manifestation of signs relative to hypovolemia do not develop until dehydration is severe (at least 8–10%). This is because for every milliliter of fluid lost from the extracellular compartment, only a fraction (usually 1/4) is lost from the intravascular compartment as compared with the fraction lost from the interstitial compartment (usually 3/4). This concept is illustrated by the example below.

6ii.1.3 Laboratory findings

After history and physical examination, clinicians can also use blood work and urinalysis (especially urine specific gravity) to assess dehydration in their patients.

Example:

A 10 kg dog who is 10% dehydrated would have effectively lost an extracellular fluid volume of 1 liter (10 kg × 0.1 = 1 l), which corresponds to 10% of its body weight. Out of those 1000 ml, that patient would have lost 750 ml from the interstitium and 250 ml from the intravascular fluid compartment.

A 250 ml decrease for this patient (assuming a vascular compartment of 80–90 ml/kg, or 800–900 ml) therefore corresponds to approximately 30% loss of circulating blood volume (250 ml / 800–900 ml = 28–31%). While compensatory mechanisms would probably also have occurred to maintain the blood volume, it can be expected that signs of hypovolemic shock would be manifested by this stage.

Blood work may show an increase in packed cell volume and/or total proteins, due to signs of hemoconcentration, or an increase in blood urea nitrogen (BUN) due to some pre-renal azotemia secondary to volume losses. As we defined clinical dehydration as isotonic fluid losses, the patient's sodium concentration should not change. If the animal loses more water than salt (hypotonic losses, for example in diabetes insipidus) or gains more water than salt is lost (in case of cardiac disease or third spacing), then the patient becomes hypernatremic or hyponatremic, respectively. Those changes will need to be addressed separately and another fluid plan created for that specific dysnatremia (see Chapter 8vi).

Urinalysis, particularly urine specific gravity, can be assessed as well, as a patient with normal kidney function should have a concentrated urine in the face of dehydration. Those changes are affected by renal values, use of diuretics or steroids, etc.

6ii.1.4 Integration of hydration assessment

Once all of these parameters are taken, they need to be integrated. The clinician will take the physical examination parameters ("6 hydration parameters"), will integrate them with history and with blood work and urinalysis findings, and will come up with a probable percentage of dehydration (% of body weight). The estimation of fluid deficit can be mild (5%), moderate (8%) or severe (10–12%). It should be remembered that the accuracy is +/– 5% for that integrated number.

6ii.2 Creating a Fluid Therapy Plan Tailored to an Individual Patient

There is technically no benefit in leaving a patient dehydrated. However, there are risks associated with overly rapid fluid administration. Also, as assessment of dehydration is not perfect, there is a risk of providing too much fluid to patients that were assessed as dehydrated, but were less than estimated or not dehydrated at all. In order to correctly and appropriately rehydrate patients, a **five-point decision-making process** can be used for actual implementation of the fluid therapy, as follows.

6ii.2.1 Fluid selection (what type?)

As dehydration has been defined as a loss of isotonic fluid, an **isotonic crystalloid** (see Chapter 3) should be chosen (Fig. 6ii.2). There are some minor differences between the various types of isotonic crystalloid (Table 6ii.2), but any kind of balanced

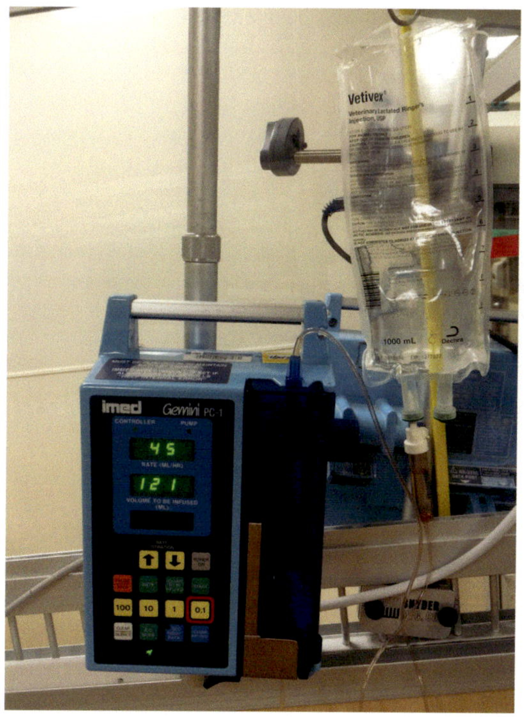

Fig. 6ii.2. Dehydration, defined as a loss of extracellular fluid compartment, is treated with an infusion of isotonic crystalloid such as lactated Ringer's solution.

Table 6ii.2. Electrolytes and buffer composition of commercially available isotonic crystalloid fluids.

	Na (mEq/l)	Cl (mEq/l)	K+ (mEq/l)	Ca++ (mEq/l)	Mg++ (mEq/l)	Buffer (mEq/l)	Buffer type	Osmolality	pH
0.9% NaCl	154	154	0	0	0	0	N/A	308	5.0
Lactated Ringer's solution™	130	109	4	3	0	28	Lactate	272	5.0
Normosol R™	140	98	5	0	3	50	Acetate Gluconate	296	6.4
pHyLyte™	140	98	5	3	0	50	Acetate Gluconate	294	7.4

electrolytes solution should be able to correct dehydration. For example, lactated Ringer's solution (LRS) is a commonly used isotonic fluid. LRS contains lactate as a buffer, as well as a small amount of calcium. Having lactate may raise questions about accuracy of lactate monitoring while administering this fluid, especially for a patient in shock. However, lactate in LRS should not be associated with a metabolic acidosis and should be metabolized within minutes if the patient has a normally functioning liver. The calcium in LRS may bind citrate contained in storage solutions in blood product, so it is recommended not to use LRS in the same line as a blood transfusion. Acetate/gluconate-buffered fluids contain no calcium but do contain magnesium. The lack of calcium and the addition of magnesium may be desirable for some clinicians, as many critical cases, especially patients with diabetes ketoacidosis, may have or develop hypomagnesemia. However, some clinicians worry that rapid intravenous administration of acetate may lead to hypotension. The authors have used both LRS and a gluconate/acetate buffered solution for fluid resuscitation in thousands of patients and have found no clinically relevant differences in resuscitation and rehydration patterns. Using 0.9% NaCl as a resuscitation and rehydration solution may lead to hyperchloremic metabolic acidosis, and a more balanced, buffered solution is usually preferred (see Chapter 3).

6ii.2.2 Volume of administration (how much?)

The amount of volume to be administered to replace dehydration is based on the degree of dehydration. As previously discussed, this will typically be assigned somewhere between 5% and 12% based on clinical assessment. As this represents the percentage of fluid lost based on body weight, the resulting volume is % dehydration (in decimal form) times body weight (kg). Therefore, a 7% dehydration on a 10 kg dog corresponds to $10 \times 0.07 = 0.7$ kg, equivalent to 0.7 l or 700 ml.

6ii.2.3 Rate of administration (how fast?)

There is considerable varying opinion regarding the optimal rate of rehydration. Usually the time-frame is 8–18 h, but it can be anywhere from 4 h to 48 h. A faster rehydration process may increase the intravascular volume and increase urine output, as the fluids do not have time to move into the interstitial compartment. This could result in less effective rehydration, or the possibility of causing volume overload. Therefore, slower rehydration plans will benefit patients with higher risks and need for closer monitoring, as clinicians need to balance risks and benefits of rehydration.

The decision about how much and how fast to give rehydration therapy may depend on several variables. In theory, patients that are very dehydrated (10–12%) can be rehydrated faster than the patients less dehydrated (5% or less). The rationale is that if a patient shows clinical signs of severe dehydration, the clinician has stronger evidence of a fluid deficit, and replacing that fluid more quickly is less risky. The chronicity of fluid loss also plays a role, as dehydration over a longer period should allow for compensatory mechanisms to take place that can be disturbed by overly aggressive fluid administration. Similarly, if compensatory mechanisms are present and the patient tolerates the fluid deficit well without changes in blood work, etc., it may be rehydrated more slowly.

The presence or absence of co-morbidity may be another major criterion affecting the creation of a fluid therapy plan and deciding on rate. Although it is very difficult to fluid overload a young and healthy patient, small animals with pre-existing heart, kidney or lung issues have higher risks of fluid overload with a rapid fluid rehydration (i.e., 4–12 h). Therefore, in patients with heart, lung and/or kidney disease, it is more prudent to rehydrate that patient over 24–48 h in more severe cases. Because of the risks associated with fluid overload, age and species also should be considered. Older patients should be rehydrated more slowly, as it may relate to higher risks of occult co-morbidity, which can be uncovered during rapid rehydration replacement. Cats should usually be rehydrated more slowly than dogs, as cats are less tolerant of large amounts of fluids than dogs.

Practicality is the other major criterion to create a fluid therapy plan. Some clinicians will rehydrate a patient overnight, others may use round numbers (e.g., 10 h or 20 h) for ease of calculation. The ability to monitor patients also plays a role in the practicality of a fluid therapy. For example, a clinician who does not have 24/7 capacity should not "plan" to have a patient rehydrated in the middle of the night and will probably choose a more gradual plan that allows reassessment the next time there are staff in the clinic. The dogma is that the more rapidly fluids are being administered, the more monitoring needs to be done, owing to the risks associated with more rapid fluid administration. Therefore, the ability to closely monitor patients should play a role in dictating the fluid therapy plan. Similarly, if a patient needs to be hospitalized for a specific amount of time (e.g., 6–12 h), then fluid therapy planning should be taken into account. Rehydration is not an exact "science", so the patient may need less (or more) of the amount of fluid calculated. Lastly, the clinician's personal preferences, knowledge of physiology and pathophysiology, and comfort level with the resulting rate may influence the speed of fluid given.

6ii.2.4 Monitoring endpoints

Normalization of hydration parameters, with body weight being the more sensitive, is the ideal endpoint. Rehydrated patients should gain an appropriate amount of weight and normalize and increase their urine output while decreasing their urine specific gravity. Patients should be carefully monitored for normalization of hydration parameters (physical examination, body weight changes, urination and thirst behavior, respiratory rate and auscultation) and blood work abnormalities (such as PCV/TP), as well as signs of fluid overload (for example, respiratory rate, physical examination findings, including development of subcutaneous edema, body weight increase above the expected number, etc.) (Mathews, 2006).

6ii.2.5 Route of administration

As the fluid deficit with dehydration usually represents a significant volume, it is usually not practical to use a subcutaneous route to provide the full rehydration volume as well as the maintenance volume. For example, a cat weighing 5 kg that is 5% dehydrated would need 250 ml (5 kg × 0.05 = 0.25 l or 250 ml) just to replace that deficit. Most clinicians would not be comfortable giving that volume to a cat. Therefore, the main route for replacing volume in dehydrated patients is ideally the intravenous route. However, if that is not an option for patient management, the clinician can decide what portion to administer. Realistically it would be challenging to give more than 2–3% of body weight by the subcutaneous route.

6ii.3 Assessing and Replacing Ongoing Losses

After calculating the maintenance rate (see Chapter 6iii) and replacement of dehydration (in this chapter), the next step is to assess and replace ongoing losses. There are various ways to assess ongoing losses, which include direct quantification or subjective assessment.

6ii.3.1 Direct measurement of losses

The best way is to accurately measure the amount of physical losses, such as vomiting, diarrhea or urinary losses, that are above normal. This is most easily accomplished when the body fluids are contained within a collection system such as with a urinary or rectal catheter, or closed-suction drain. Quantification of losses can also be achieved by weighing disposable pads containing urine or liquid feces/vomit. Once the weight of the pad itself is subtracted, the remaining weight should equate to the volume of fluid (1 g = 1 ml).

Strong documentation of ongoing losses in medical records, as well as strong communication with the nursing team, is important. Losses can be assessed at regular time intervals, such as every 4–12 h, and then have the volume replaced over the time it was lost.

Example:

A patient urinates into a disposable pad. The total weight is 90 g, and it is known that the pad itself weighs 40 g. It can therefore be determined that the weight or volume of urine is 50 g or 50 ml (90 g – 40 g = 50 g).

Example:

If it appears that a patient has lost 120 ml of fluid over the past 6 h, then 20 ml/h should be added for the next 6 h of scheduled fluid therapy (120 ml / 6 h = 20 ml/h).

This precise way can be best used on cases of post-obstructive diuresis after de-obstruction of a cat with urethral obstruction, or for a polyuric recovery phase of acute renal failure.

6ii.3.2 Estimation of losses

Most clinicians will replace ongoing losses using an arbitrary value, which traditionally has been based on the maintenance rate, setting the rate at 1.5–2 times the calculated value. In this regard, the clinician will pre-emptively provide a little more fluid than calculated with the maintenance and replacement of losses, with the expectation that the patient will continue to have losses, usually in the form of vomiting and/or diarrhea. This practice works well for most patients hospitalized for vomiting and/or diarrhea. If the patient's renal function is intact, the kidneys would be able to balance the needs of the body to maintain homeostasis and the fluid provided by the clinician if the patient was receiving more than was needed. In addition, monitoring as described above can allow the clinician to determine if further adjustment is needed.

6ii.4 Conclusion

In conclusion, replacing fluid volume in dehydrated patients, which is the basis of treatment of various

Clinical Case 6ii.1

A 6-year-old male castrated Beagle (20 kg) presents with non-specific clinical signs including lethargy and inappetence, with two bouts of vomiting.

On physical examination, he is assessed as between 5% and 10% dehydrated (so you will pick 8% for the calculations).

Owners declined workup but agreed to overnight hospitalization. It is currently 4pm and the owner is picking up the patient at 8am tomorrow morning. You therefore have 12–16 h to rehydrate this dog.

First determine the approach to the fluid deficit (dehydration).

Fluid type:

The fluid deficit is from the extracellular fluid compartment, so it is isotonic fluid loss that should be replaced by an isotonic crystalloid. Plasma-Lyte A is chosen.

How much:

It was determined that the patient is 8% dehydrated. The calculation is as follows:

20 kg × 0.08 = 1.6 l, so 1600 ml deficit.

How fast:

The deficit can be replaced safely between 10 h and 24 h. However, because you have a limited amount of time in which the patient is hospitalized, the recommendation would be 12–16 h. Because the volume to be replaced is 1600 ml, an easy way is to replace it over 16 h, as it gives you a nice round number of 100 ml/h and does not require the use of a calculator.

Please note that 12 h is not wrong either, in which case the rate would be 133 ml/h.

Then, calculate the maintenance fluid rate.

What type:

For ease most clinicians will use the same isotonic fluid that is being used for rehydration. A hypotonic fluid could also be used. See Chapter 6iii for more information.

How much/how fast:

It is decided to use the allometric scale, so a maintenance rate of 132 × $BW^{0.75}$ (kg) per day is selected. This results in a maintenance rate of 52 ml/h that should be added to the deficit/dehydration volume.

Contribution of ongoing losses:

At this stage it is not known what the extent of ongoing losses will be. While half of maintenance (26 ml/h) could be added as an estimate, it is decided to wait and attempt to quantify the losses.

Integration and final starting rate:

The final fluid therapy plan should be 100 ml/h (dehydration) + 52 ml/h (maintenance) = 152 ml/h for 16 h, then discharge patient.

diseases and very commonly done in hospitalized patients, requires a basic understanding of physiology, some clinical skills, and a systemic approach to the patient, as well as making an educated guess to create and monitor a fluid therapy plan. There are three main components that need to be incorporated to determine the **overall replacement rate:**

$$\% \text{ dehydration} \times \text{body wt/(hours of replacement)} + \text{ongoing losses/h} + \text{maintenance rate}$$

The next section (Chapter 6iii) will discuss the application of this last component—maintenance rate and fluid therapy—to round out the general approach to fluid administration.

The two case examples will apply the principles of replacement fluid therapy discussed in this chapter. Case information has been kept limited to reduce distractions. However, they represent cases commonly seen in practice.

Clinical Case 6ii.2

You are presented with a 3-year-old 50 kg Saint-Bernard with profuse diarrhea with blood and vomiting. The dog got into the garbage a couple of days ago, so you suspect a case of hemorrhagic gastroenteritis, also known as acute hemorrhagic diarrhea syndrome. Physical examination shows severe dehydration with hypovolemia, so you assume your patient is probably 10% dehydrated. Minimum database shows hemoconcentration (PCV 70%, TP 6.0 g/dl), which confirms your suspicion of severe dehydration.

Given these findings, hospitalization and supportive care are strongly recommended, to which the owner agrees.

First determine the approach to the fluid deficit (dehydration).

Which type:

The fluid deficit is from the extracellular fluid compartment, so isotonic fluid loss that should be replaced by an isotonic crystalloid. A decision for Normosol R is made.

How much:

Assuming 10% deficit on a 50 kg dog the calculation is as follow: 50 × 0.10 = 5.0 l, so 5000 ml. This "feels" like a large volume, but you are dealing with a large dog who is severely dehydrated and hemoconcentrated. Trust your calculations.

How fast:

There are two main options that are commonly used in a clinical setting.

The first option is to correct this dehydration fairly quickly (6–8 h) as your patient has severe dehydration with signs of hypovolemia. Based on this your rate would be 625 ml/h over 8 h or 833 ml/h over 6 h. Most clinicians will pick a round number within that range that corresponds to their clinical style; 700–800 ml/h would be reasonable.

After 6–8 h, the fluid rate should be dropped to maintenance + ongoing losses (see below). Again, those numbers may seem high, but should be safe in this patient with no known co-morbidities. With this type of rapid rehydration, the patient should be frequently reassessed for signs of fluid overload (increased respiratory rate, crackles, etc.) during the first 6–8 h.

The second option is to give a fluid bolus at admission, using an isotonic fluid that will redistribute between the intersitium and the intravascular compartments: maybe 1000 ml over 30 min to correct the hypovolemia (see Chapter 6i for more information). Because your deficit is 5000 ml and you already gave 1000 ml as a bolus, now you must give only 4000 ml for dehydration. You can correct it around 8–12 h, which is 330–500 ml/h.

Then, calculate the maintenance fluid rate.

Which type:

Most clinicians will use the isotonic fluid that is being used for rehydration.

How much/how fast:

Using the allometric scale with $132 \times BW^{0.75}$ (kg) per day, the maintenance fluid is 103 ml/h that should be added to the deficit/dehydration volume (Davis *et al.*, 2013).

Contribution of ongoing losses:

As the patient is more likely to continue to have ongoing losses, it is prudent to add some additional volume to the fluid therapy plan, between 0.5 to 1× maintenance, so 50–100 ml/h. If there is concern regarding the overall rate, it may be reasonable to wait and carefully monitor/quantify *actual* losses (i.e., vomiting and diarrhea) and adjust accordingly.

Integration and final rate determination:

- **Option 1:** 700 ml/hr for 7 h (dehydration) + 100 ml/h (maintenance), so 800 ml/h for 7 h, then 200 ml/h (maintenance with ongoing losses).
- **Option 2:** 1000 ml over 30 min, then 600 ml/h for 8 h (deficit 500 ml/h + 100 ml/h for maintenance), then 200 ml/h (maintenance with ongoing losses).

It is important to note that with either option the same amount of fluid will have been given after 24 h and the patient should be adequately rehydrated. The decision depends mainly on physical examination findings and the risks and benefits of the different fluid rates, as well as clinical style, your staffing and facility, and the amount of time the owner will give to treat.

References

Davis, H., Jensen, T., Johnson, A. *et al.* (2013) 2013 AAHA/AAFP fluid therapy guidelines for dogs and cats. *Journal of the American Animal Hospital Association* 49(3),149–159.

DiBartola, S. and Bateman, S. (2006) Introduction to fluid therapy. In: DiBartola, S.P. (ed.) *Fluid, Electrolyte and Acid-Base Disorders in Small Animal Practice*. Saunders Elsevier, St Louis, Missouri, pp. 325–344.

Mathews, K. (2006) Monitoring fluid therapy and complications of fluid therapy. In: DiBartola, S.P. (ed.) *Fluid, Electrolyte and Acid-Base Disorders in Small Animal Practice*. Saunders Elsevier, St Louis, Missouri, pp. 377–391.

Wellman, M., DiBartola, S. and Kohn, C. (2006) Applied physiology of body fluids in dogs and cats. In: DiBartola, S.P. (ed.) *Fluid, Electrolyte and Acid-Base Disorders in Small Animal Practice*. Saunders Elsevier, St Louis, Missouri, pp. 3–26.

6iii Maintenance Fluid Therapy

Jiwoong Her

The Ohio State University, Columbus, Ohio, USA

The term "maintenance" in fluid therapy has three different meanings. **Maintenance phase** is typically the last phase among the three phases of fluid therapy (resuscitation, replacement, and maintenance). In chronological order, this phase usually begins no sooner than 12–24 h after fluid therapy has begun. At this time point, the patient has been resuscitated to compensate for shock (resuscitation phase), and then received adequate amounts of fluid as a full or partial replacement of estimated fluid deficit (replacement phase). **Maintenance rate (requirement)** refers to the estimated volume of fluid to maintain normal physiological losses (urine, feces, evaporation, etc.). It is administered in conjunction with fluid to replenish fluid deficit and pathologic ongoing losses (vomiting, diarrhea, excessive urination, etc.) to preserve fluid balance during the maintenance phase. **Maintenance fluid** refers to the type of fluid resembling normal physiologic fluid losses. Physiologic losses are relatively low in sodium and high in potassium compared with plasma or commercial replacement solutions. Therefore, maintenance fluids are usually hypotonic crystalloids that contain a higher amount of potassium and lower sodium compared with plasma. Further details of these three concepts will be discussed throughout this chapter.

6iii.1 Maintenance Phase

Fluid therapy is divided into three phases: resuscitation phase (see Chapter 6i); replacement phase (see Chapter 6ii); and maintenance phase. The maintenance phase is typically the last phase of fluid therapy. Objective signs indicating that the patient is ready to be placed in the maintenance phase are the absence of clinical signs of shock as well as full/partial replacement of estimated fluid deficit. These signals can be evaluated by six perfusion parameters to assess the intravascular compartment (mentation, mucous membrane color, capillary refill time, pulse quality, pulse rate, and distal extremity temperature) and six hydration parameters to assess interstitial compartment (moistness of mucous membrane, skin elasticity, eye position, changes in body weight, thirst, and signs of hypovolemia). During the maintenance phase, patients receive fluid therapy only to meet daily maintenance requirement.

6iii.2 Maintenance Rate (Requirement)

Maintenance rate is defined by the volume of fluid needed per day to keep the patient in zero fluid balance (no net gain or loss). In other words, it is to replace physiologic losses when the patient is hospitalized and withheld from food and water (Silverstein and Santoro-Beer, 2015). The two categories that contribute to maintenance rate include sensible and insensible losses. Approximately two-thirds of the maintenance rate are sensible losses and one-third is insensible loss. In classic definition, a **sensible loss** is the loss that can be perceived by the senses, which include urine, feces, and saliva. In practical terms, sensible loss is a measurable water loss mainly by urine, because it is usually impractical to measure losses via feces or saliva (unless there is a significant increase in GI losses, such as diarrhea, but these would then no longer be considered maintenance). Furthermore, urine is the most important predictable sensible loss in healthy dogs and cats (typically 1–2 ml/kg/h). **Insensible loss** (difficult to measure) refers to the amount of fluid lost through other routes, such as respiratory tract and skin. This type of loss is not easily measured, because it is mainly evaporative loss of electrolyte-free water. In humans, approximately two-thirds of the insensible losses occur by evaporation of water from the skin. In contrast, dogs and cats under normal conditions have minimal water loss via skin, because sweat glands do not actively participate in the central thermoregulatory mechanism (Wellman *et al.*, 2012). As discussed, in practical terms, insensible losses also include water lost in

DOI: 10.1079/9781789243406.0063

the feces and saliva, which are difficult to measure.

Daily maintenance rate can be calculated in several ways in dogs and cats (Table 6iii.1). Most formulas are based on the estimations obtained in laboratory settings where healthy animals are housed under conditions mimicking hospitalized sick patients (DiBartola and Bateman, 2012). Daily fluid requirement for healthy dogs with minimal activity in ambient temperature is proportional to their energy requirement at the rate of 1 kcal = 1 ml. Several studies have reported a wide range of daily maintenance rates in dogs (48–183 ml × $BW_{kg}^{0.75}$).

Table 6iii.1. Commonly suggested formulas for maintenance fluid requirements.

Dog and cat	70 × $(BW_{kg})^{0.75}$/day (30 × BW_{kg} + 70)/day 40–60 ml/kg/day
Dog	132 × $(BW_{kg})^{0.75}$/day 2–6 ml/kg/h
Cat	70–80 × $(BW_{kg})^{0.75}$/day 2–3 ml/kg/hr
Neonate/pediatric	80–120 ml/kg/day 3-4 ml/kg/h

Table 6iii.2. BCS scales and their relationship with body fat (BF) and body weight (BW). (Adapted from Cline *et al.*, 2021.)

9-point scale	5-point scale	% BF	% Overweight
4	2.5	15–19	Ideal[a]
5	3	20–24	
6	3.5	25–29	10%
7	4	30–34	20%
8	4.5	35–39	30%
9	5	40–45+	40%
> 9	> 5		> 40%

[a] Ideal body weight (assuming 20% BF) = Current body weight × (100 – %BF)/0.8

Adult cats have lower daily fluid requirement than dogs, for multiple reasons, including: lower blood volume per kilogram; lower ratio of water to caloric needs (0.6–0.7:1 in cats versus 1:1 in dogs); and greater ability to concentrate urine. The authors' intensive care unit uses daily maintenance rate of 132 ml × $BW_{kg}^{0.75}$ and 80 ml × $BW_{kg}^{0.75}$ [a] as a starting point for dogs and cats, respectively. These exponential equations were found to give more accurate estimates of true requirements across all body weights, whereas linear equations will underestimate or overestimate the requirements for animals that are smaller (< 3–5 kg) or larger (> 25 kg), respectively (DiBartola and Bateman, 2012). Lastly, it is recommended to calculate fluid requirements based on ideal body weight to avoid overhydration, especially in patients with obesity, because fat has a lower water content than lean mass. American Animal Hospital Association Weight Management Guidelines suggest the estimation of the ideal weight using body condition score (BCS) scale for dogs and cats (Table 6iii.2) (Cline *et al.*, 2021).

It is important to note that the true maintenance rate varies significantly between patients. In addition, it may be altered significantly in a patient depending on ambient temperature, the level of activity, age, or disease process. For example, a patient with excessive panting will lose a larger amount of electrolyte-free water by respiratory evaporation. Young patients will require greater volumes of fluid than adults, due to their larger ratio of surface to body mass (see Chapter 8viii). Patients with certain illnesses such as diabetes insipidus, diabetes mellitus, hyperadrenocorticism, kidney disease, etc. may have increased urinary losses from decreased concentrating ability, thereby requiring a higher "maintenance" fluid rate. Daily fluid requirement is also affected by composition of the patient's diet (wet food versus dry food). Therefore, no single approach can precisely estimate maintenance requirement for each patient.

Table 6iii.3. Composition of commonly available hypotonic crystalloids compared with plasma.

		Electrolyte (mEq/l)					Buffer (mEq/l)				
Fluid	pH	Na+	Cl-	K+	Ca^{2+}	Mg^{2+}	Lactate	Acetate	Gluconate	Osmolality (mOsm/l)	Glucose (g/l)
0.45% NaCl	5.0	77	0	77	0	0	0	0	0	154	0
0.45% NaCl with 2.5% dextrose	4.5	77	0	77	0	0	0	0	0	280	25
Plasma-Lyte 56 in 5% dextrose	5.0	40	40	13	0	3	0	16	0	363	50
Normosol-M in 5% dextrose	5.0	40	40	13	0	3	0	16	0	363	50
5% Dextrose	4.0	0	0	0	0	0	0	0	0	252	50
Plasma	7.4	142	104	5	5	3	0	0	0	300	

Regardless of the calculation chosen, serial evaluation of the patient's fluid balance is the most important aspect of providing a fluid rate tailored to the individual patient's requirement.

Estimation of maintenance requirement in Table 6iii.1 does not include hydration status of the patient or pathological ongoing losses (vomiting, diarrhea, excessive urination, etc.). Therefore, replacement of the hydration deficit and ongoing losses must be considered in conjunction with the daily maintenance requirement (see Chapter 6ii). Six hydration parameters can be used to assess dehydration (see Chapter 6ii). Ongoing losses can be a very important component of fluid therapy, though it may be difficult to accurately predict the amount of fluid lost in vomitus or diarrhea. Excessive urine output can be replaced ("ins and outs") by either placing a urinary catheter in a closed collection system or weighing bedding to estimate voided urine (1 g = 1 ml urine voided). In a clinical setting, repeated assessment of patient body weight may provide a reliable way to determine net gain or loss (e.g., 1 kg = 1 l = 1000 ml of gain or loss). The authors' intensive care unit measures body weight at least once daily, or more frequently in critically ill patients.

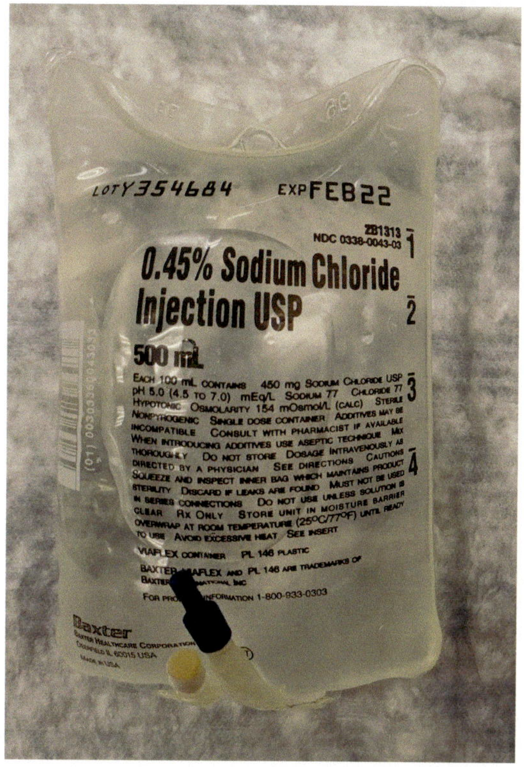

Fig. 6iii.1. An example of a hypotonic fluid: 0.45% NaCl.

6iii.3 Maintenance Fluid

In general, crystalloids are categorized as being hypertonic, isotonic, or hypotonic based on effective osmolarity in relation to plasma osmolality (see Chapter 3). Crystalloids also can be classified as replacement (isotonic) or maintenance (hypotonic) fluids. **Isotonic fluids** (e.g., Normosol-R, Plasma-Lyte 148) are intended to be used to replace lost body fluids and electrolytes during the resuscitation or replacement phase, because they are largely restricted to the extracellular fluid compartment upon administration. **Maintenance fluids** (e.g., Normosol-M, Plasma-Lyte 56, 0.45% NaCl) are hypotonic crystalloids that contain a lower amount of sodium, and may have a higher amount of potassium compared with plasma, which more closely resembles physiologic losses (Fig. 6iii.1). These hypotonic fluids distribute throughout the total body water (both intracellular and extracellular compartments), leaving relatively lower amounts in the extracellular space. Therefore, maintenance fluids are indicated to replace normal ongoing losses of patients during the maintenance phase in which water intake is restricted, or the losses are not beyond normal physiologic losses. In addition, these can be used to replenish free water deficits in patients with hypotonic or pure water loss. For patients who have impaired excretion of sodium (kidney disease) or decreased tolerance to an elevated intravascular volume (cardiac disease), maintenance fluids are a safer choice, due to the larger volume of distribution and lower sodium load.

Maintenance fluids exist in many compositions. Table 6iii.3 details the composition of commonly available maintenance fluids. The major differences between maintenance fluids are the composition of electrolytes and type of buffer contained within the fluid. Thus, fluid selection will depend on the acid–base and electrolyte status of the patient. Half-strength saline (0.45% NaCl) is an excellent maintenance fluid. It can be combined with maintenance dose (e.g., 20 mEq/l) of potassium chloride (see Chapter 7ii) and 2.5–5% dextrose (see Chapter 7i). If commercial maintenance fluids are not readily available, they can be formulated in-house by mixing 5% dextrose to isotonic fluids (for example, 0.9% NaCl, Plasma-Lyte 148, or lactated Ringer's solution) at a 1:1 ratio. The simplest formula is to mix 500 ml of D5W (dextrose 5% in water) into 500 ml of 0.9% NaCl, which makes 1 l of 0.45% saline with 2.5% dextrose. Another example: mixing one part (333 ml) 0.9% NaCl with two parts (666 ml) 5% dextrose and adding 20 mEq potassium chloride makes 1 l of fluid with 51 mEq/l sodium, 20 mEq/l potassium, 71 mEq/l chloride, and 33.5 g/l dextrose. Its osmolality is 328 mEq/kg providing 133 kcal/l.

Most maintenance fluids contain dextrose in order to increase the osmolality of the fluid. Glucose increases the osmolality of the fluid *in vitro*, which brings the osmolality into an isotonic range for infusion. Once administered, the glucose is quickly oxidized to carbon dioxide and water by cells, which reduces the tonicity of fluid. To summarize, a bag of maintenance fluid containing dextrose is iso-osmolar as it is administered but becomes effectively hypotonic once the dextrose is metabolized. Without the addition of dextrose to maintenance fluids, these could have a dangerously low tonicity, particularly for rapid infusion (Lanaux, 2018). Therefore, maintenance fluids (hypotonic fluids) should never be administered as bolus therapy or used for intravascular volume resuscitation. Rapid infusion of hypotonic fluids causes sudden shifts of water from the extracellular space into the intracellular space, causing hemolysis or cellular swelling (cerebral edema). It is worth noting that the presence of 2.5–5% dextrose in these fluids supplies only a few percentages of daily energy requirements.

The major buffers in commercial maintenance fluids include lactate, acetate, and gluconate. These are bicarbonate precursors which consume hydrogen ions during metabolism, yielding an alkalinizing effect. These buffered fluids are selected to treat metabolic acidosis. The pH of these fluids is usually acidic (4.0–5.0,) due to the presence of dissolved carbon dioxide and dextrose in the solutions. However, the total quantity of free hydrogen ions in these fluids is small and easily buffered *in vivo*, and therefore is of little clinical significance. Further discussion of the effects of various fluids on the acid–base disturbances can be found in Chapter 3.

Clinicians often use replacement fluid (isotonic fluid) during maintenance phase to replenish estimated fluid deficit and daily maintenance requirement. Using replacement fluid for the short-term maintenance phase typically does not alter electrolytes significantly, because patients with normal kidney function can excrete excess water or electrolytes. However, long-term administration of isotonic fluid during the maintenance phase may lead to electrolyte imbalance, especially in patients with renal or cardiac disease. There is ongoing debate regarding the merits of isotonic versus hypotonic fluids as maintenance fluid therapy in both human and veterinary medicine (Hansen and Vigani, 2017). From the viewpoint of providing daily requirements to maintain net zero fluid balance, the ideal maintenance fluid is hypotonic which resembles the physiologic electrolyte losses. However, excessive

Clinical Case 6iii.1

A 2-year-old, 45 kg MC Labrador with BCS 9/9 is presented to your clinic for elective orthopedic surgery scheduled tomorrow. He is normally hydrated with no known ongoing losses. Food and water will be withheld from the patient during hospitalization overnight. How much intravenous fluid should be given?

Ideal body weight (assuming 20% body fat) = Current body weight × (100 – %BF)/0.8 = 45 kg × (1.0–0.4) /0.8 = 33 kg
Maintenance rate = 132 × $(33)^{0.75}$/24 h = 75 ml/h (maintenance-type fluid)

Please note the difference compared with the calculation based on the patient's actual weight:

Maintenance rate = 132 × $(45)^{0.75}$/24 h = 96 ml/h (maintenance-type fluid)

This patient would receive 20 ml/h (or almost 500 ml/day) more than he needs.

Clinical Case 6iii.2

A 5-year-old 10 kg mixed-breed dog has been treated with isotonic crystalloid for chronic diarrhea. On day 3, diarrhea is resolved, and the dog continues to have decreased appetite. This morning the patient is assessed to be euhydrated. How much fluid should be given during the next 24 h?

Volume of fluid required = fluid deficit (estimated zero) + maintenance volume + ongoing loss (assumed zero)
Maintenance volume = 132 × $(10)^{0.75}$/day = 31 ml/h
Total 31 ml/h of maintenance-type fluid (e.g. 0.45% NaCl) over the next 24 h

Clinical Case 6iii.3

A 2-year-old, 5 kg, domestic shorthaired cat is being treated for urethral obstruction. The cat was resuscitated on presentation, followed by replacement of the deficit volumes over the past 12 h. Now you are faced with a euhydrated cat with post-obstructive diuresis. The urine output measured via urinary catheter over the past 4 h was 200 ml. How much fluid will you give over the next 4 h?

Total = fluid deficit (estimated zero) + maintenance (insensible losses + sensible losses) + ongoing losses

Insensible losses = 22 ml/kg/day = 4.6 ml/h

Note: It is important not to include the entire maintenance rate in addition to the urinary losses. As urine output accounts for most of the normal maintenance, this would essentially result in giving that volume twice.

Urine output (200 ml/4h) = sensible loss + ongoing loss = 50 ml/h

Total = 54.6 ml/h (4.6 ml/h of maintenance-type fluid and 50 ml/h of replacement-type fluid) over the next 4 h.

However, given that the insensible loss is relatively negligible compared with the urinary losses, to approximate and match the urine output would be reasonable (50 ml/h).

administration of hypotonic fluids may lead to water retention and subsequently hyponatremia, which is associated with poor outcomes in dogs and cats. A recent Cochrane review in children recommended isotonic over hypotonic fluid for maintenance fluid therapy, due to its protective effect against hyponatremia (Mcnab *et al.*, 2014). On the other hand, excessive administration of isotonic fluids may lead to sodium retention and volume overload, which has a strong negative impact on outcome. Frequent monitoring of volume status and electrolyte changes is recommended to optimize patient outcome. Eventually, maintenance fluid therapy can be discontinued when the patient can maintain fluid balance on its own by adequate oral intake of food and water.

References

Cline, M.G., Burns, K.M., Coe, J.B. *et al.* (2021) 2021 AAHA weight management guidelines for dogs and cats. *Journal of the American Animal Hospital Association* 50(1), 1–11.

DiBartola, S.P. and Bateman, S. (2012) Introduction to fluid therapy. In: DiBartola, S.P. (ed.) *Fluid, Electrolyte, and Acid-Base Disorders in Small Animal Practice*, 4th edn. W.B. Saunders, St Louis, Missouri, pp. 331–350.

Hansen, B. and Vigani, A. (2017) Maintenance fluid therapy: isotonic versus hypotonic solutions. *Veterinary Clinics: Small Animal Practice* 47(2), 383–395.

Lanaux, T. (2018) Maintenance fluid therapy. In: Drobatz, K.J., Hopper, K., Rozanski, E. and Silverstein, D.C. (eds) *Textbook of Small Animal Emergency Medicine*. Wiley Online Books, John Wiley & Sons, Hoboken, New Jersey, pp. 1132–1135.

McNab, S., Ware, R.S., Neville, K.A. *et al.* (2014) Isotonic versus hypotonic solutions for maintenance intravenous fluid administration in children. *Cochrane Database of Systematic Reviews* 12, CD009457.

Silverstein, D.C. and Santoro-Beer, K. (2015) Daily intravenous fluid therapy. In: Silverstein, D.C. and Hopper, K. (eds) *Small Animal Critical Care Medicine*, 2nd edn. W.B. Saunders, St Louis, Missouri, pp. 316–321.

Wellman, M.L., DiBartola, S.P. and Kohn, C.W. (2012) Applied physiology of body fluids in dogs and cats. In: DiBartola, S.P. (ed.) *Fluid, Electrolyte, and Acid-Base Disorders in Small Animal Practice*, 4th edn. W.B. Saunders, St Louis, Missouri, pp. 2–25.

7i Dextrose Supplementation

Edward Cooper

The Ohio State University, Columbus, Ohio, USA

While the previous chapters have been geared toward the various types, routes, and rates of fluid administration, sometimes fluid therapy alone is not sufficient to replenish electrolyte or metabolic deficiencies. In these circumstances it is necessary to provide additional sources of supplementation to meet these needs. This chapter will focus on the most common additives (dextrose, potassium, calcium, phosphorus, and magnesium) used in various clinical circumstances, with an emphasis on indications for use and the associated calculations to make sure delivery is able to meet the patient's needs safely. First will be consideration of dextrose supplementation.

7i.1 Glucose Utilization and Regulation

Glucose is a breakdown product of carbohydrate metabolism and feeds into cellular energy production as the main substrate for glycolysis. The end product of glycolysis is pyruvate, which then sets the stage for the Krebs cycle and eventually oxidative phosphorylation. The resulting generation of ATP provides the energy source for various functions and maintenance of cellular homeostasis. While alternate energy sources (like fatty acids) can also drive this process, some cells (e.g., red blood cells and neurons) are almost exclusively dependent on glucose. Maintenance of a normal blood glucose level is therefore essential and the development of hypoglycemia constitutes a life-threatening emergency.

There are a number of hormones in the body that can affect the blood glucose. **Insulin** is essentially the only substance in the body that functions to decrease blood glucose. Released from the pancreatic beta cells in response to hyperglycemia, insulin triggers the activity of glucose transporters and the associated intracellular shift. Glucose is then metabolized, turned into fatty acids, or stored as glycogen. It is important to note that glucose transport in neurons is not insulin dependent, but rather concentration dependent. This means that glucose uptake into neurons is entirely a function of blood/interstitial glucose concentration.

While insulin serves to decrease blood glucose, there are several counter-regulatory hormones that function to increase blood glucose: catecholamines, cortisol, glucagon, and growth hormone. **Catecholamines and glucagon** are released as the most immediate response to decreases in blood glucose. They help to increase blood glucose by stimulating glycogenolysis and gluconeogenesis (Cryer and Arbeldez, 2020). Catecholamines do this both directly and by facilitating the effects of glucagon. **Cortisol** promotes the mobilization of amino acids and fatty acids to serve as alternate energy sources. **Growth hormone** also promotes lipolysis (Cryer and Arbeldez, 2020). All four of the counter-regulatory hormones antagonize the effects of insulin and decrease peripheral glucose utilization.

7i.2 Causes of Hypoglycemia

Given the extensive system designed to maintain blood glucose, it becomes apparent that hypoglycemia can only occur when these mechanisms are absent, overwhelmed or become exhausted. Categorically this can occur with excessive insulin (endogenous or exogenous) or insulin-like factors, decreased glucose production, increased glucose consumption, drug-associated, or spurious. See Box 7i.1 for a more detailed list, and other resources for more detailed descriptions (Forcada, 2017; Gonzalez and Silverstein, 2019).

7i.3 Clinical Signs and Diagnosis

The principal manifestation of hypoglycemia is related to the central nervous system. As previously mentioned, glucose transport in the brain is dependent on a concentration gradient rather than insulin. A decrease in blood glucose will then cause a

DOI: 10.1079/9781789243406.0071

Box 7i.1. Select causes of hypoglycaemia.

Excess insulin or insulin-like factors

- Exogenous insulin overdose
- Functional beta cell tumor (insulinoma)
- Paraneoplastic
    - Hepatocellular carcinoma/hepatoma
    - Leiomyosarcoma/leiomyoma
    - Lymphoma
    - Hemangiosarcoma

Increased glucose consumption

- Sepsis
- Hunting dog hypoglycemia
- Pregnancy

Decreased glucose production

- Hypoadrenocorticism
- Hepatic disease
    - Acute hepatic failure
    - Portosystemic shunt
- Neonates/pediatrics/toy breeds

Drug-associated

- Xylitol
- Beta-blockers

Spurious

- Polycythemia/leukocytosis
- Analytical delay/equipment error

significant reduction in available intracellular glucose concentration. This, combined with the high neuronal metabolic demand, leads to rapid depletion of energy stores and disruption of cellular function. The result is a process called **neuroglycopenia**—essentially hypoglycemia of the brain—which can be associated with a variety of clinical signs (Loose *et al.*, 2008). The initial response reflects sympathetic activation: restlessness, agitation, muscle tremors, shaking, tachycardia. This progresses to more overt neurological dysfunction: lethargy, ataxia, seizures, and eventual coma.

Concern for hypoglycemia based on presentation for seizures or other neurological signs, especially in conjunction with, for example, a known history of diabetes/insulin administration, neonates/pediatrics, xylitol exposure, etc., should prompt measurement of blood glucose. A value less than 60 mg/dl with associated clinical signs and a clinical response to dextrose administration fulfills Whipple's triad for diagnosis of hypoglycemia (Cryer and Arbeldez, 2020). While this seems straightforward, there are factors that can complicate diagnosis. Hand-held glucometers can have variable accuracy and so validation of findings might be needed if there is disparity with the clinical picture (Cohen *et al.*, 2009). It is also important to remember that samples can have falsely low blood glucose measurements if analysis or separation of serum from the red blood cells is not performed promptly. Red blood cells will continue to metabolize glucose as the sample sits, potentially resulting in an incorrect diagnosis of hypoglycemia. In addition, there may be a disconnect between the blood glucose measurement and clinical signs. While it is typically expected that neurological signs will develop with a blood glucose below 50 mg/dl, patients with chronic hypoglycemia (e.g., insulinoma or chronic insulin overdose) may need to reach a much lower value (< 20–30 mg/dl).

Any further diagnostic evaluation of the hypoglycemic patient is geared toward determining the underlying cause. Signalment, history, pertinent physical examination findings, and any abnormalities on screening blood work (complete blood count, biochemical profile) should narrow the differential list and inform diagnostic selection (such as abdominal imaging, resting cortisol, insulin levels, etc.).

7i.4 Treatment

Once the presence of hypoglycemia has been established (or is highly suspected) in the symptomatic patient, treatment should be instituted immediately. In these circumstances it is important to increase blood glucose rapidly by administration of a dextrose bolus. The recommended dose is typically 0.25–0.5 g/kg, given IV or IO. Dextrose often comes as a 50% (0.5 g/ml) stock solution (Fig. 7i.1), so this works out as 0.5–1.0 mL/kg which must be diluted 1:2 or 1:3 with sterile water or an isotonic crystalloid and delivered over 5 min. This is necessary given the very hypertonic nature of the stock solution and the potential to cause severe phlebitis. Historically the practice of applying karo syrup or dextrose solution to the gums to promote mucosal absorption has been used for patients at home, or when IV/IO access cannot be obtained. However, it has been shown that transmucosal absorption is not effective, and oral administration only works if the solution is swallowed (Gunning and Garber, 1978).

It is generally expected that clinical signs will improve within minutes of administration if hypoglycemia was responsible for the clinical signs. However, severe neuroglycopenia can result in persistent signs and delayed neurologic recovery even after the blood glucose has been normalized. Care must also be taken with administration of a dextrose bolus to patients with suspected insulinoma. A sudden increase in blood glucose can trigger massive release of insulin from the functional beta-cell tumor, thereby resulting in a rapid return to hypoglycemia. For this reason, a dextrose bolus should not be given to automatically treat a low blood glucose unless the patient is overtly clinical. In addition, smaller boluses of dextrose (0.1–0.2 g/kg) should be considered so that just enough is given to reverse or improve clinical signs and limit the stimulation of insulin release. For patients with highly suspected or a confirmed diagnosis of insulinoma, administration of glucocorticoids and/or glucagon may be warranted to limit the potential for this vicious cycle.

If a dextrose bolus was necessary to address clinical signs, then a continuous rate infusion (CRI) will likely be needed. This will also be the case for hypoglycemic patients that are not yet clinical but expected to become clinical in the near future (e.g., pediatrics or insulin overdose). A dextrose CRI is typically given as a 2.5–5.0% solution by adding the 50% stock solution to the patient's IV fluids (see Clinical Case 7i.1 for example calculations). The decision of whether to use 2.5% or 5% is somewhat subjective. For mild to moderate hypoglycemia, 2.5% is often chosen with the option to increase to 5% if that does not adequately support blood glucose. If supplementation greater than 5% is needed, ideally a central catheter should be placed to limit the degree of vascular irritation caused when hyperosmolar solutions are administered peripherally.

7i.5 Monitoring and Discontinuing Supplementation

Blood glucose should be monitored after beginning supplementation, with frequency dictated by how dynamically changes are expected (typically every

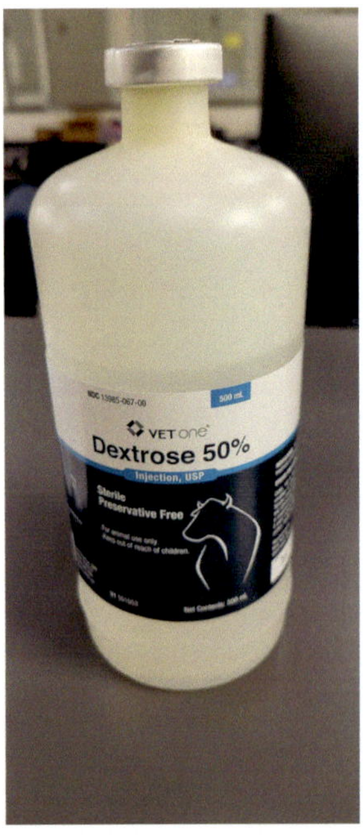

Fig. 7i.1. An example of 50% dextrose stock solution.

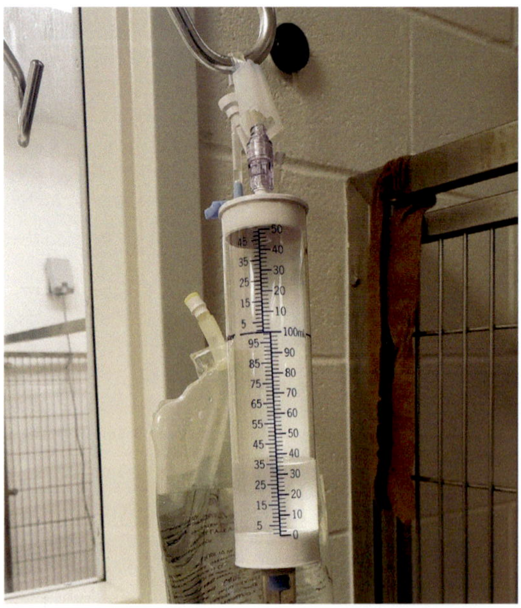

Fig. 7i.2. Example of a buretrol which allows supplementation of a smaller volume at a time.

Clinical Case 7i.1

You have an 8 kg 6-year-old Miniature Schnauzer previously diagnosed as diabetic that has presented for having accidentally received a double dose of insulin this morning. He had become progressively lethargic then started seizuring just before he arrived. On initial assessment the dog is now minimally responsive, twitching and found to have a blood glucose of 42 mg/dl. An IV catheter is placed, and it is decided to give a 0.5 g/kg dextrose bolus from a 50% (0.5 g/ml) stock solution:

Dose: 0.5 g/kg × 8 kg = 4 g
Volume: 0.6 g ÷ 0.5 g/ml = 4 ml

Based on this, 4 ml of 50% dextrose is then combined with 8 ml of sterile water to achieve a 1:2 dilution. The volume is given over 5 min. It is then decided to create a 2.5% dextrose CRI using a 500 ml bag of lactated Ringer's solution which will provide the patient's fluid therapy. Here is how you determine the calculation.

The best approach to calculating dilutions is to use:

$$V_1 \times C_1 = V_2 \times C_2$$

where

V_1 = volume of stock solution – ?
C_1 = concentration of stock solution – 50%
V_2 = final desired volume – 500 ml
C_2 = final desired concentration – 2.5%

The volume of 50% dextrose needed is the only unknown, so the equation is rearranged:

$$V_1 = V_2 \times C_2/C_1$$
$$= 500 \text{ ml} \times 2.5\%/50\%$$
$$= 25 \text{ ml}$$

Ideally, 25 ml would be removed from the bag of LRS and then add 25 ml of 50% dextrose to achieve a 2.5% solution (though practically the 25 ml of dextrose could be just added to the bag). The blood glucose is rechecked 2 h later and found to be only 51 mg/dl. It is decided to increase to 5% dextrose solution. Since he may need frequent adjustments to his supplementation, you elect to switch to using a 100 ml buretrol. To make a 5% solution:

$$V_1 = V_2 \times C_2 / C_1$$
$$= 100 \text{ ml} \times 5\%/50\%$$
$$= 10 \text{ ml}$$

Based on this calculation, 10 ml of 50% dextrose is added to 90 ml of LRS in the buretrol for a total of 100 ml of a 5% dextrose solution. After 6 h of dextrose supplementation his blood glucose is now 240 mg/dl so you are comfortable with decreasing back to 2.5%. After another 4 h his blood glucose is 302 g/dl and so his dextrose is stopped.

2–8 h). If the need for frequent measurements is expected, placement of a sampling catheter/central line is recommended to decrease imposition on the patient and the nursing team. If this is not possible, other options to minimize the impact include the use of an insulin syringe or repeated use of an ear prick site. The target of dextrose supplementation is not necessarily to normalize blood glucose, but rather to maintain an acceptable level that is not associated with any clinical signs (typically at least 60 mg/dl). For smaller patients that might need frequent adjustments, use of a buretrol allows for modulation of a smaller volume (rather than changing the whole fluid bag). See Fig. 7i.2 for an example.

The decision to decrease or discontinue dextrose supplementation can depend on several factors. If the underlying cause of hypoglycemia has been addressed, treated, or resolved, it would be reasonable to trial a reduction or removal of dextrose from the fluids altogether. Certainly, if the patient becomes hyperglycemic the amount of dextrose should be decreased. However, it is important to note that patients with a normally functioning pancreas will not necessarily develop hyperglycemia in the face of unneeded supplementation. Along those lines, a patient with a normal blood glucose may or may not still need to be on dextrose. In these circumstances the only way to make that determination is to decrease or turn off the dextrose infusion and monitor blood glucose closely. If levels are maintained, then further reduction or discontinuation is warranted.

References

Cohen, T.A., Nelson, R.W., Kass, P.H. *et al.* (2009) Evaluation of six portable blood glucose meters for measuring blood glucose concentrations in dogs. *Journal of the American Veterinary Medical Association* 235, 276–280.

Cryer, P.E. and Arbeldez, A.M. (2020) Hypoglycemia. In: Melmed, S., Auchus, R.J., Goldfine, A.B., Koenig, R.J. and Rosen C.J. (eds) *Williams Textbook of Endocrinology*, 14th edn. Elsevier, Philadelphia, Pennsylvania, pp. 1525–1551.

Forcada, Y. (2017) Hypoglycemia, hyperglycemia. In: Ettinger, S.J., Feldman, E.C. and Cote, E. (eds) *Textbook of Veterinary Internal Medicine*, 8th edn. Elsevier, St Louis, Missouri, pp. 246–249.

Gonzalez, A.L. and Silverstein, D.C. (2019) Hypoglycemia. In: Drobatz, K.J., Hopper, K., Rozanski, E. and Silverstein, D.C. (eds) *Textbook of Small Animal Emergency Medicine*, John Wiley and Sons, Hoboken, New Jersey, p. 719.

Gunning, R.R. and Garber, A.J. (1978) Bioactivity of instant glucose. Failure of absorption through oral mucosa. *Journal of the American Medical Association* 240(15), 1611–1612.

Loose, N.L., Rudloff, E. and Kirby, R. (2008) Hypoglycemia and its effect on the brain. *Journal of Veterinary Emergency and Critical Care* 18, 223–234.

7ii Potassium Supplementation

PAGE YAXLEY

The Ohio State University, Columbus, Ohio, USA

7ii.1 Potassium Function

Potassium is the major intracellular cation, with 95% or more of total body potassium located within the cell and only 5% in the extracellular fluid (ECF). Potassium concentration is 140 mEq/l in the intracellular fluid (ICF), as compared with 4 mEq/l in the extracellular fluid. Intracellular potassium is important for the maintenance of normal cell volume, and is required for normal enzyme function, as well as DNA, glycogen, and protein synthesis (DiBartola, 2012). Perhaps the most important function is generating normal resting cell membrane potential and regulating the function of depolarizable tissue (cardiac, skeletal muscle, nerves) (DiBartola, 2012; Odunayo, 2014).

Potassium is critically maintained within narrow limits to avoid the life-threatening effects of hypokalemia or hyperkalemia. The balance between the ECF and the ICF is maintained by the sodium–potassium adenosine triphosphatase (ATPase) pump. During normal homeostasis, the sodium–potassium ATPase pump drives sodium ions out of the cell and potassium in at a 3:2 ratio (Phillips and Polzin, 1998; DiBartola, 2012) (Fig. 7ii.1). The cumulative effect is a higher intracellular to extracellular ratio of potassium resulting in a negative electrical gradient or resting membrane potential (RMP). A cell reaches threshold membrane potential when sodium entry exceeds potassium exit (DiBartola, 2012). Depolarization allows nerve conduction and muscle contraction. Cell excitability is directly related to the difference between RMP and threshold potential, therefore the smaller the difference between these two, the more excitable the cell (Phillips and Polzin, 1998; DiBartola, 2012).

7ii.2 Potassium Balance

Balance of potassium is maintained normally by matching loss (urine) to intake (diet). Potassium enters the body unregulated through the gastrointestinal tract (Phillips and Polzin, 1998; DiBartola, 2012). All ingested potassium is absorbed in the stomach and small intestine, where transport of potassium is passive. Colonic absorption of potassium is active (DiBartola, 2012).

Once ingested, potassium is rapidly redistributed into the intracellular space under the influence of catecholamines (beta-2 adrenergic) and insulin (Phillips and Polzin, 1998; DiBartola, 2012) (Fig. 7ii.1). Endogenous insulin secretion enhances uptake of potassium and promotes cellular entry independent of glucose uptake. Stimulation of beta-2 adrenergic receptors by epinephrine promotes cellular uptake of potassium in liver and muscle by increasing the activity of the cell membrane sodium–potassium ATPase pump. As excess ingested is excreted, potassium is gradually released back into the extracellular space.

Potassium is predominantly removed from the body through the kidneys (urine 90–95% removal) and to a lesser extent by the gastrointestinal tract (5–10%). Renal excretion of potassium load occurs primarily through glomerular filtration, alterations in proximal tubular reabsorption, and distal tubular secretion. The efficiency of this system is crucial to prevent life-threatening hyperkalemia.

7ii.3 Normal Serum Concentrations

Normal serum concentrations vary slightly amongst dogs and cats and laboratories but are expected to be 3.5–5.5 mEq/l, averaging 4.5. Any changes that arise in serum potassium concentrations must arise from a change in one of the following: (i) intake; (ii) distribution/transcellular shift; or (iii) excretion (Phillips and Polzin, 1998; DiBartola, 2012; Odunayo, 2014).

DOI: 10.1079/9781789243406.0072

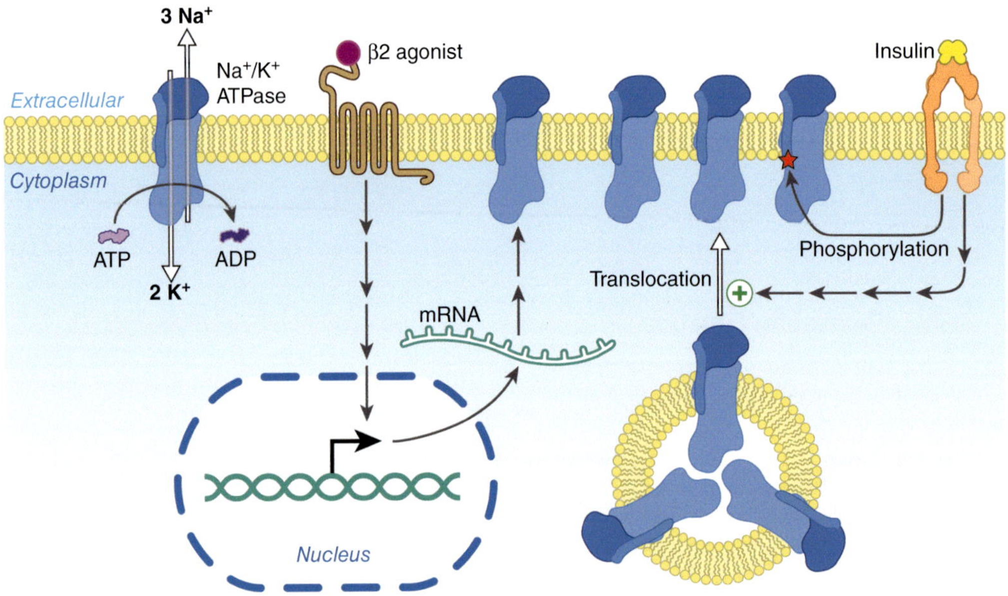

Fig. 7ii.1. Graphic depiction of the sodium potassium ATPase pump. Hormonal influence from insulin and B2 activation is also depicted. (© The Ohio State University.)

7ii.4 Hyperkalemia

Hyperkalemia is associated most commonly with decreased excretion (Table 7ii.1). However, other causes, including altered distribution and increased intake, are possible, though less likely if renal and adrenal function are normal (Odunayo, 2014). **Pseudohyperkalemia** is a term used when there is *in vitro* release of intracellular potassium and does not reflect true *in vivo* levels. **Hyperkalemia** is defined as serum concentration exceeding 5.5 mEq/l and is considered life threatening when concentrations are > 7.5 mEq/l. Severe hyperkalemia requires rapid correction to prevent cardiovascular collapse (Odunayo, 2014).

Hyperkalemia makes the RMP less negative, bringing the RMP and threshold membrane potential closer together. As the cell becomes more excitable, prolonged de- and repolarization of the myocardial conduction system may occur. Clinically, bradycardia is most commonly noted (Phillips and Polzin, 1998; Odunayo, 2014). If the RMP drops below threshold membrane potential, the cell depolarizes but cannot repolarize. Arrhythmias arise in a predictable and recognizable pattern with tall, tented t-waves, prolonged PR interval, sinoatrial block, widened QRS complexes, atrioventricular conduction blocks, ventricular fibrillation, and asystole (Fig. 7ii.2). While these changes generally worsen as serum potassium increases, the ECG cannot predict potassium level, and vice versa. As such, it is possible that the ECG can be normal with life-threatening hyperkalemia (Odunayo, 2014). Cardiac effects may also be aggravated by hyponatremia, hypoglycemia, and acidosis (Phillips and Polzin, 1998).

7ii.4.1 Treatment of hyperkalemia

The goal of treatment of hyperkalemia is to correct and prevent cardiovascular collapse (see Table 7ii.2 for an overview of medications used in the treatment of hyperkalemia). Calcium gluconate provides cardioprotection by restoring the potential difference between the RMP and the threshold membrane potential (Odunayo, 2014). Calcium gluconate (10%) dosed at 50–100 mg/kg IV is administered slowly over 5–10 min. Due to risk of bradycardia and asystole, heart rate monitoring with an ECG is recommended. The cardioprotective effects begin immediately and are anticipated to last 30–60 min (Odunayo, 2014). It is important to note that calcium gluconate does not serve to reduce the

Table 7ii.1. Causes of hyperkalemia (adapted from Odunayo (2014) to reflect the most clinically relevant).

Presentation	Potential causes
Decreased excretion	Anuric/oliguric renal failure Cavitary effusions Drugs (ACE inhibitors, potassium sparing diuretics) Hypoadrenocorticism Uroabdomen Urethral obstruction Whipworms
Altered distribution (translocation to the ECF)	Massive tissue damage Reperfusion injury Metabolic acidosis Nonspecific beta blockers
Pseudohyperkalemia	Thrombocytosis

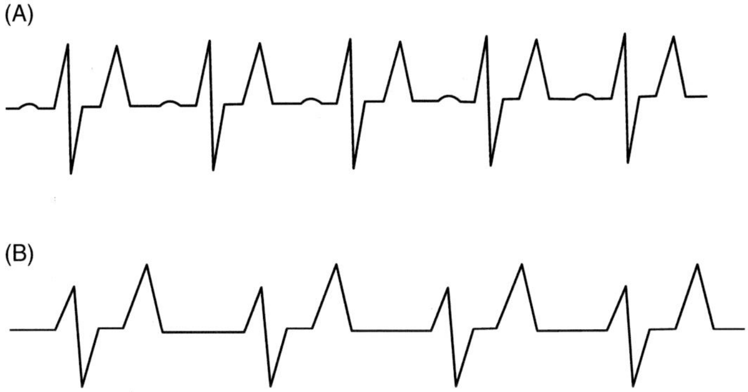

Fig. 7ii.2. Potential ECG changes associated with (A) moderate (approx. 6.0–8.0 mEq/l) and (B) severe hyperkalemia (> 8.0 mEq/l).

Table 7ii.2. Emergency dosing for severe hyperkalemia. All medications are given intravenously.

Medication	Dose	Rate of administration	When to administer
Calcium gluconate	50–100 mg/kg	3–5 min	Bradycardia, major ECG changes
Regular insulin	0.25 u/kg	IV bolus	If Ca gluconate given Potassium > 8 mEq/l
Dextrose	0.5 g/kg	3–5 min	If regular insulin given Potassium > 8 mEq/l
Terbutaline	0.01 mg/kg	IV bolus	If Ca gluconate given Potassium > 8 mEq/l
Sodium bicarbonate (used uncommonly)	1 mEq/kg	5 min	Potassium> 10 mEq/l pH < 7.0

potassium level itself, and so other interventions are needed before the protective effect is lost.

To aid in redistribution of ECF potassium into the ICF, clinicians can administer regular insulin at a dose of 0.25 u/kg IV. Insulin will promote a shift of potassium into cells about 15 min after administration and will likely last 2–4 h. It is advisable to concurrently administer dextrose (0.5g/kg IV), as insulin will also redistribute glucose intracellularly (Odunayo, 2014). As the effects of insulin might extend beyond the duration of the dextrose bolus, blood glucose levels should be checked in

30–60 min, and dextrose supplemented as needed. While sole administration of dextrose has been touted to induce endogenous insulin release, the results are inconsistent (Odunayo, 2014).

Beta-2 adrenergic agonist (such as terbutaline) may be considered as an adjunct treatment, driving potassium intracellularly by increasing sodium–potassium ATPase activity (Odunayo, 2014). Terbutaline can be given at 0.01 mg/kg IV. The effects of beta-2 adrenergics usually start within 30 min and can last 2 h (Odunayo, 2014).

Sodium bicarbonate has also been used to redistribute potassium to the intracellular space. Due to its delayed onset of action, the risk of metabolic alkalosis, hypernatremia and paradoxical CNS acidosis, and the availability of other safer options, sodium bicarbonate is rarely used (Odunayo, 2014).

Fluid therapy can also be helpful in the treatment of hyperkalemia. Isotonic crystalloid therapy including 0.9% sodium chloride (containing no potassium), and potassium-containing fluids (lactated Ringer's solution, Plasma-Lyte A, Normosol-R) can be administered safely as long as the underlying reason for hyperkalemia is concurrently being treated (Dibartola, 2012; Odunayo, 2014). Volume expansion will enable dilution. The effect again will begin immediately and may require hours to be most effective (Odunayo, 2014). In patients that are oliguric/anuric, fluids containing potassium should be avoided.

The most effective way to reduce hyperkalemia remains diversion of urine. This can be accomplished through urethral catheterization if the patient has a urethral obstruction, decompressive cystocentesis, or through abdominal draining in the event of a uroabdomen. This can also be achieved more aggressively through hemo- or peritoneal dialysis (Odunayo, 2014). The latter may have limited availability for the acute hyperkalemic crisis and may be prohibitively expensive. The onset of action to reduce hyperkalemia with urinary diversion will likely require 1–5 h to have significant effect (Odunayo, 2014).

7ii.5 Hypokalemia

Hypokalemia is arguably the most commonly encountered electrolyte abnormality in veterinary medicine and is found in 20% of hospitalized human adults (Gennari, 1998; Odunayo, 2014). Hypokalemia is defined as serum potassium less than 3.5 mEq/l. Similarly, potassium depletion may be due to increased excretion, redistribution or inadequate intake (DiBartola, 2012; Odunayo, 2014) (Table 7ii.3).

While tolerated in most patients, symptoms can correlate to rapidity of the decrease in potassium level, with the most profound effects seen when serum levels get below 2.0–2.5 mEq/l (Gennari, 1998; Odunayo, 2014). **Hypokalemic polymyopathy**

Table 7ii.3. Causes of hypokalemia (adapted from Odunayo (2014) to reflect the most clinically relevant).

Presentation	Potential causes
Increased excretion	Gastrointestinal disorders Aldosterone-secreting tumor Chronic kidney disease Diabetic ketoacidosis Post-obstructive diuresis Diuretic therapy (furosemide, thiazides, acetazolamide) Mineralocorticoids (fludrocortisone) Renal tubular acidosis type I and II Hyperadrenocorticism
Altered distribution (translocation to the ICF)	B adrenergic therapy or intoxication (albuterol, terbutaline) Theophylline Hyperthyroidism Insulin administration Metabolic alkalosis Refeeding syndrome Hypokalemic periodic paralysis (Burmese cats)
Inadequate intake	Administration of potassium-free fluids Severely potassium-deficient diet Prolonged anorexia

(Fig. 7ii.3) is a term used to describe severe skeletal muscle weakness, often clinically noted as severe ventroflexion of head and neck, stiff gait, plantigrade stance, respiratory arrest from diaphragmatic and/or respiratory muscle failure (Phillips and Polzin, 1998; Odunayo, 2012). Potentially fatal effects of hypokalemia are usually related to disturbances in cardiac electrical cavity. Reduced extracellular potassium concentrations make the RMP more negative, thereby decreasing excitability and prolonging repolarization. Delayed and abnormal repolarization increase automaticity, and increase duration of the action potential. Reported ECG changes include ST segment depression and decreased T-wave amplitude, formation of U waves, and prolonged PT intervals (Phillips and Polzin, 1998). This in turn predisposes the patient to atrial and ventricular tachyarrhythmias, atrioventricular dissociation, and ventricular fibrillation (Odunayo, 2014).

Potassium depletion also impairs potassium metabolism during muscle contraction and exercise, resulting in ischemia (Phillips and Polzin, 1998). Rhabdomyolysis has been reported with severe hypokalemia (Odunayo, 2014). Hypokalemia reduces renal blood flow and glomerular filtration, potentially contributing to renal vasoconstriction, especially in cats. Polyuria and polydipsia may clinically manifest, due to impaired thirst and urine-concentrating mechanism associated with hypokalemia. Hypokalemia has been linked to decreased renal responsiveness to ADH (Phillips and Polzin, 1998) and may worsen hepatic encephalopathy by promoting increased production of ammonia.

Potassium and magnesium also have a unique relationship (Gennari, 1998). Magnesium depletion, due to reduced intake or abnormal loss, reduces the intracellular potassium concentrations and causes renal potassium wasting in humans. This is thought to be associated with an impairment of the activity of the cell membrane sodium–potassium ATPase pump, but the complete mechanism is unclear. Regardless of cause, the ability to correct potassium deficiency is impaired when magnesium deficit is present (particularly if it is < 0.5 mmol/l) (Gennari, 1998). Clinicians should evaluate and consider supplementation of magnesium in refractory hypokalemic patients (see Chapter 7iv for more information).

7ii.5.1 Treatment of hypokalemia

The goal of treatment of hypokalemia is to prevent or correct cardiac electrical disturbances and serious muscle weakness. The long-term goal is to return total body potassium concentrations to normal and identify and treat underlying disease (Odunayo, 2014).

Potassium can be supplemented parenterally or enterally. Options for parenteral supplementation include potassium chloride (KCl at 2 mEq/ml) and potassium phosphate (K_2HPO_4 or KH_2PO_4 at 4.4 mEq/ml) (DiBartola, 2012). Potassium chloride is preferred to also support concurrent chloride depletion if vomiting or diuretic administration is the underlying cause of hypokalemia. Supplementation of potassium should be calculated rather than estimated (DiBartola, 2012).

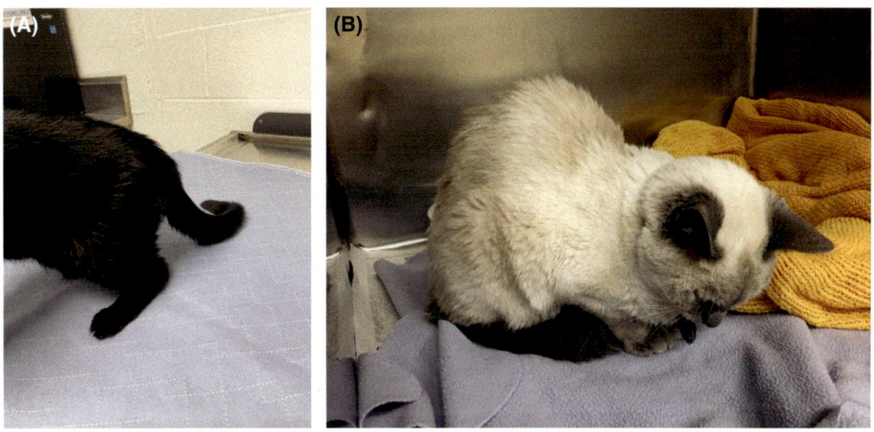

Figure 7ii.3. Depiction of **(A)** severe plantigrade stance and **(B)** cervical ventroflexion in cats with severe hypokalemia. (Images courtesy of Jessica Quimby, DVM, PhD, DACVIM.)

Commonly, potassium supplementation is added to isotonic crystalloid fluid therapy using standard dosing charts (Table 7ii.4). Infusion of potassium-containing fluids may initially result in a decrease in potassium concentration in measured serum, as a result of dilution and increased cellular uptake (DiBartola, 2012). Increased distal renal tubular flow may also transiently reduce measured potassium levels. It is important to mix thoroughly after potassium supplementation is added to a fluid bag, to prevent inadvertent high concentration of potassium being pulled into the fluid line (DiBartola, 2012). Care should be taken to avoid phlebitis and sclerosis of peripheral veins, and therefore it is recommended not to exceed 60 mEq/l unless a central line is used. Parenteral fluids containing up to 35 mEq/l KCl have been safely administered subcutaneously (DiBartola, 2012). Mild to moderate hypokalemia may not adequately resolve on lower fluid rates; likewise, higher fluid rates may cause hyperkalemia with supplementation (Odunayo, 2014). With higher fluid rates or fluid potassium concentration, care should be taken not to exceed the maximum rate of supplementation, i.e., 0.5 mEq/kg/h (K_{max}), to avoid development of iatrogenic hyperkalemia and potential for adverse cardiac effects. This can be determined based on potassium concentration in the fluids, fluid rate, and patient weight. See Clinical Case 7ii.1 for example calculations. It is important to note that patients with severe dehydration or renal dysfunction may have a reduced K_{max} owing to impaired excretion.

In critically ill patients, or patients with dynamic fluid requirements, more precise correction of potassium may be required. If an animal has normal renal function, intravenous replacement rates with continuous rate infusion of 0.1–0.5 mEq/kg/h delivered by syringe pump can be used depending on the severity of the hypokalemia (see Clinical Case 7ii.2). This approach can also be helpful if it is thought that there will be frequent changes to fluid rate or potassium supplementation (such as with DKA). Again, dose should not exceed 0.5 mEq K/kg/h (K_{max}). At the author's institution, if concurrent administration of intravenous fluids is at least at a maintenance rate, potassium is diluted 1:2 with sterile water, placed on a syringe pump, and attached to a port nearest the patient to minimize the amount of concentrated potassium in the line. If no additional fluid therapy is being concurrently administered, then it is diluted 1:4 with sterile water and is delivered through a peripheral line, or 1:2 if delivered through a central line. Serial monitoring will be necessary (see section 7ii.5.2 below).

Careful potassium supplementation is important when using insulin to treat patients with diabetic ketoacidosis (DiBartola, 2012). This condition is associated with a chronic depletion of total body potassium. At presentation, serum potassium is often normal to increased, because of lack of insulin. Marked hypokalemia can develop with the resolution of hyperglycemia, and concurrent use of insulin therapy. For this reason, insulin or sodium bicarbonate administration should be delayed for 2–4 h after initiating rehydration, and serum potassium levels have been replenished (DiBartola, 2012; Odunayo, 2014).

Oral potassium supplementation is preferred in patients that can tolerate it and is considered safer, because the potassium enters circulation much more slowly (Gennari, 1998). Potassium gluconate is preferred, due to palatability. Potassium citrate, which also offers increased palatability, may ameliorate metabolic acidosis (Phillips and Polzin, 1998; DiBartola, 2012). Oral potassium supplementation is common in patients with chronic kidney disease or other causes of chronic hypokalemia and is occasionally used to reduce calcium oxalate urolithiasis. Various supplements are available. Dosing

Table 7ii.4. Potassium Supplementation Chart ("Sliding Scale of Scott"). Recommendations based on patient being placed on a maintenance fluid rate.

Patient serum K levels (mEq/l)	Suggested K supplementation (mEq/l)	Resulting K concentration (mEq/ml)	Equivalent K CRI rate (mEq/kg/h)
3.5–5	20	0.02	0.1
3–3.4	30	0.03	0.2
2.5–2.9	40	0.04	0.3
2–2.4	60	0.06	0.4
< 2	80	0.08	0.5

should be based on manufacturer's label and titrated in response to therapy (Odunayo, 2014).

7ii.5.2 Monitoring

Serial measurements of potassium should be conducted during supplementation or in patients at high risk of developing potassium disorders (DiBartola, 2012). Frequent vomiting, diarrhea, polyuria, muscle weakness, unexplained arrhythmias, or where the patient is receiving insulin, supplemental potassium, total parenteral nutrition or diuretic therapy should prompt monitoring (Kogika and Morais, 2008). Frequent monitoring (every 6–8 h) of serum potassium concentration is recommended when aggressive replenishment is required (Odunayo, 2014). In hospitalized patients, if sampling from a line, a three-syringe technique is recommended to prevent inadvertent error. The amount of supplementation must be determined through serial measurements of serum potassium concentrations during treatment and recovery (DiBartola, 2012).

Clinical Case 7ii.1

A 5-year-old, 15 kg male castrated mixed-breed dog presents for 3 days of vomiting and diarrhea. The patient is found to be 8% dehydrated, but is cardiovascularly stable (fluid resuscitation is not needed). It is decided to replace the dehydration over 12 h, as well as provide maintenance requirement, using an isotonic crystalloid (Plasma-Lyte). The resulting fluid rate is 140 ml/h (see Chapter 6ii for information on how this was determined). The patient also has a potassium level of 2.9, and so it is decided to add KCl at 40 mEq/l to the fluid bag. Prior to starting, the rate of potassium administration is calculated to make sure it is below K_{max}:

Plasma-Lyte contains K at 5 mEq/l, so need to add 35 mEq KCl to achieve 40 mEq total
40 mEq/l = 0.04 meq/ml (40 mEq/l/1000 ml)
Rate of potassium administration (mEq/h) = fluid rate × K mEq/l = 140 × 0.04 = 5.6 mEq/h
Rate of potassium administration (mEq/kg/h) = mEq/h / wt(kg) = 5.6/15 = 0.37 mEq/kg/h
Rate of potassium administration < Kmax, administration should be safe

As the potassium rate is below K_{max}, it is safe to add 35 mEq of KCl which has a concentration of potassium of 2 mEq/ml. To calculate the amount of KCl to add:

Dose desired/stock concentration = 35 mEq/2 mEq/ml = 17.5 ml KCl added to 1 l Plasma-Lyte

What if there was only 800 ml (0.8 l) left in the bag? The calculation would need to be adjusted:

17.5 mL KCl added to 1 l, so need to multiply by 0.8 to determine amount:
17.5 × 0.8 = 14 ml KCl added to 800 ml Plasma-Lyte

Clinical Case 7ii.2

Your 5 kg feline patient has been diagnosed with diabetic ketoacidosis. After initial fluid resuscitation it is decided to start potassium supplementation, the patient's potassium level currently being 3.1 mEq/l. In anticipation of needing to make frequent changes to the rate of potassium supplementation, it is decided to use a CRI at 0.2 mEq/kg/h. The infusion will be going through a peripheral catheter with concurrent fluids, so a 1:2 dilution is used. You decide to make 6 h-worth of solution, and so have the following calculations:

0.2 mEq/kg/h × 5 kg = 1.0 mEq/h
1 mEq/h × 6 h = 6 mEq KCl needed
6 mEq / 2 mEq/ml = 3 ml of KCl

To make a 1:2 dilution:

3 ml KCl added to 6 ml of sterile water for a total volume of 9 ml

To determine the new concentration:

C2 = (C1 × V1)/V2 = (2 × 3)/9 = 0.67 mEq/ml

Syringe pump set to 0.2 mEq/kg/h, weight 5 kg, concentration 0.67 mEq/l

References

DiBartola, S.P. (2012) *Fluid, Electrolyte, and Acid-Base Disorders in Small Animal Practice*, 4th edn. Elsevier Saunders, St Louis, Missouri.

Gennari, F.J. (1998) Hypokalemia. *New England Journal of Medicine* 339(7), 451–458.

Kogika, M.M. and de Morais, H.A. (2008) Hypokalemia: a quick reference. *Veterinary Clinics of North America: Small Animal Practice* 38, 481–484.

Odunayo, A. (2014) Management of potassium disorders. *Clinician's Brief* March, 69–72.

Phillips, S.L. and Polzin, D.J. (1998) Clinical disorders of potassium homeostasis: hyperkalemia and hypokalemia. *Veterinary Clinics of North American: Small Animal Practice* 28(3), 545–564.

7iii Calcium and Phosphorus Supplementation

ANDA YOUNG

The Ohio State University, Columbus, Ohio, USA

The regulation of calcium (Ca) and phosphorus (Pi) is coordinated by an orchestra of hormones and effector organs (Fig. 7iii.1). Parathyroid hormone (PTH) can be thought of as the conductor giving cues to organ systems including the kidneys, bone, intestinal tract, and parathyroid glands to perform a specific function that ultimately leads to minute-to-minute alterations in calcium and phosphorus levels. Additionally, PTH interacts with other major regulators of calcium homeostasis such as calcitriol (activated vitamin D) and calcitonin (produced in thyroid as C cells). The goal of this section will be to briefly review the regulation of calcium and phosphorus homeostasis, pathologic aberrancies, and approaches to clinical supplementation. An exhaustive review of calcium and phosphorus homeostasis can be found elsewhere (DiBartola and Willard, 2012a,b).

7iii.1 Hormonal Regulation of Calcium

Calcium is predominantly stored in bone (99%) with the remaining 1% being stored in extracellular spaces in complexed, protein-bound, and ionized forms (DiBartola andf Willard, 2012a). Calcium is vital to a multitude of biological roles in the body, including muscle contraction, vascular tone, coagulation, hormone secretion, glycogen metabolism, hormone secretion, enzymatic activity, neurotransmitter release, and nerve cell membrane stabilization (DiBartola and Willard, 2012a). Too much or too little of this divalent cation may lead to severe consequences in sensory-somatic processes. As such, the body exercises strict control over fluctuations of ionized calcium levels.

The parathyroid glands are small glands located on the rostral and caudal aspects of the right and left thyroid lobes that function as "calciostatic" organs (Bergwitz and Juppner, 2010). The pea-sized parathyroid glands house chief cells that are responsible for sensing circulating ionized calcium (iCa) levels through an iCa-sensing receptor and responding appropriately through production, release, and degradation of PTH. Low levels of PTH are secreted continuously to maintain normal serum iCa levels (DiBartola and Willard, 2012a). Sensation of hypocalcemia leads to an upregulation of PTH release and a net effect of increased serum iCa levels and a decrease in serum phosphate levels (Bergwitz and Juppner, 2010).

Hypocalcemia leads to biphasic release of stored PTH; initial release occurs within seconds and remains enhanced minutes to hours later. Other stimulators of enhanced PTH release include mild hyperphosphatemia, catecholamines, and mild to moderate hypomagnesemia (Molina, 2018). On the contrary, **hypercalcemia** inhibits PTH secretion via enhanced intracellular PTH degradation. Hypercalcemia, as sensed by iCa-receptors, leads to degradation of up to 90% of preformed PTH within chief cells. This negative feedback mechanism is relied on when diagnosing primary hyperparathyroidism versus other sources of hypercalcemia (e.g., hypercalcemia of malignancy). Other inhibitors of PTH release include hypophosphatemia, vitamin D, and severe hypomagnesemia (paradoxical block) (Molina, 2018).

PTH binds to parathyroid hormone receptors in proximal renal tubular epithelial cells where it stimulates 1α-hydroxylase, converting inactive calcidiol/25$(OH)_2$D to active calcitriol/1,25$(OH)_2$D. Calcitriol will then circulate to enhance Ca and Pi levels in circulation through effects on the intestine, bone, and kidneys. Calcitriol will negatively feedback on PTH release and 1α-hydroxylase enzymes acting as a checks-and-balance system, blunting excessive levels of Ca and Pi (DiBartola and Willard, 2012a,b).

DOI: 10.1079/9781789243406.0073

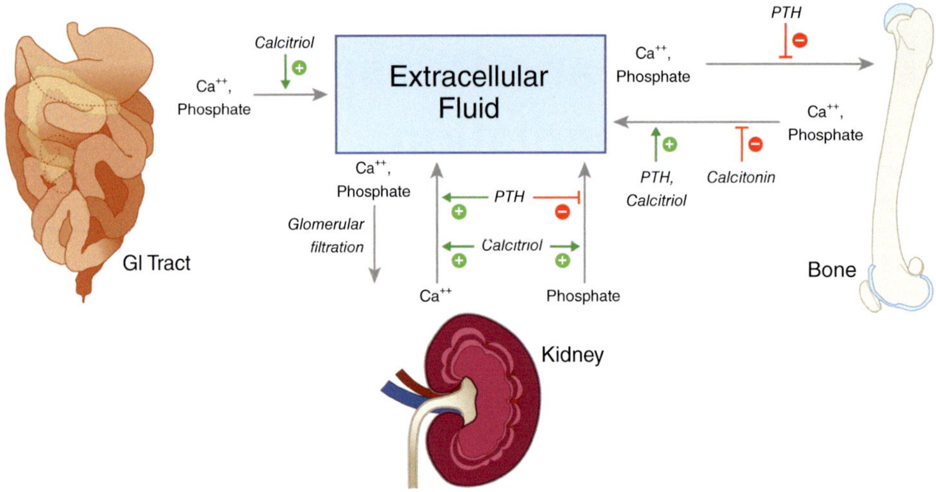

Fig. 7iii.1 Hormonal influences on kidney, bone, and intestinal tract alter serum calcium and phosphorus levels through effects of reabsorption/secretion, resorption, and absorption, respectively. (© The Ohio State University.)

7iii.2 Hormonal Regulation of Phosphorus

Phosphate is predominantly stored in bone (80–85%) and soft tissue cells (15%) with only 1% residing in serum and extracellular fluids (Huang *et al.*, 2013). Phosphate participates in structural and functional roles as a component for bony hydroxyapatite, nucleic acids, signaling molecules, phospholipids, and co-factors for cellular metabolism (DiBartola and Willard, 2012b).

PTH facilitates phosphate excretion in the proximal tubule through internalization and degradation of apical type II $Na^+PO_4^{2-}$ co-transporters (Molina, 2018). As PTH can be thought of as a "phosphaturic" hormone, fibroblast growth factor-23 (FGF23) is considered a historical "phosphatonin" whose role in phosphorus regulation should not be underemphasized. FGF23 is an endocrine hormone mainly produced by osteoblasts and osteocytes in response to hyperphosphatemia and calcitriol. The principal action of FGF23 is suppression of proximal tubule phosphate reabsorption using mechanisms previously mentioned, including Na/Pi co-transporter internalization and degradation. Oppositional to PTH, FGF23 suppresses activity of 1α-hydroxylase, preventing vitamin D activation, which blunts intestinal absorption of phosphorus (Erben, 2018). In chronic kidney disease, it becomes relevant that hyperphosphatemia and subsequent increased levels of FGF23 suppress calcitriol, leading to loss of PTH inhibition and the phenomenon of renal secondary hyperparathyroidism (Dittmer *et al.*, 2017).

7iii.3 Parathyroid Hormone Effector Organs

PTH has direct effects on the kidneys and bone while having indirect effects on the intestinal tract (Fig. 7iii.1). Under the influence of PTH there is a global effect of increased serum ionized calcium via increased renal reabsorption, increased bone resorption, and increased intestinal absorption through the effects of calcitriol.

In the kidney, PTH performs three major functions, including enhanced Ca^{2+} reabsorption, phosphorus excretion, and stimulation of 1α-hydroxylase, leading to generation of the active vitamin D metabolite, calcitriol. Calcium reabsorption is facilitated by PTH-mediated Ca^{2+} channel insertion in the apical membrane of the distal tubule. Once intracellular, cytosolic diffusion of Ca^{2+} is facilitated by a vitamin D-dependent carrier protein known as calbindin-D28k. Reabsorption then occurs through basolateral Ca^{2+}/Na^+ exchangers and CaATPase efflux pumps (Molina, 2018).

In bone, PTH-mediated osteoblast activation precedes osteoclastic activation and Ca/Pi liberation. Once activated, osteoclasts attach to bone surface generating an acidic, enzyme-rich microenvironment that facilitates the breakdown of hydroxyapatite and subsequent Ca/Pi liberation (Molina, 2018).

In the intestinal tract calcium is absorbed via passive paracellular (non-saturable) and active transcellular routes (saturable), with the latter being calcitriol dependent. Mechanisms of Ca^{2+} entry mimic that of the kidney such that calcium channels facilitate intracellular entry, calbindin mediates transcellular transport (calcitriol mediated), followed by active efflux of Ca^{2+} mediated by Ca^{2+}ATPase and Na^{+}/Ca^{2+} exchangers (Molina, 2018). Efforts to prevent postprandial hypercalcemia are largely regulated by the hormone calcitonin. Calcitonin secretion is enhanced from thyroid C cells in response to hypercalcemia or following a calcium-rich meal. Calcitonin functions to inhibit osteoclastic action; however, its effects are transient and considered to be a minor contributor in calcium homeostasis.

7iii.4 Causes of Alterations in Calcium and Phosphorus

The pathophysiology of hypercalcemia, hypocalcemia, hyperphosphatemia, and hypophosphatemia in veterinary patients has been recently reviewed (Allen-Durrance, 2017; de Brito Galvão *et al.*, 2017a,b; Gonzales, 2018). A recent retrospective study described calcium derangements, correlating severity as it relates to etiology (Coady *et al.*, 2019) (Figs 7iii.2 and 7iii.3).

The most common cause of **hyperphosphatemia** in dogs and cats is decreased excretion secondary to acute kidney injury and/or chronic renal disease (Allen-Durrance, 2017). Other mechanisms of elevated phosphate levels include cellular translocation (e.g., tumor lysis syndrome, trauma, metabolic acidosis), increased intestinal absorption (e.g., phosphate enemas, vitamin D toxicosis), growth stages, and laboratory error (DiBartola and Willard, 2012b). **Hypophosphatemia** is commonly seen secondary to cellular translocation (e.g., insulin therapy, respiratory alkalosis/hyperventilation, malnourishment/refeeding syndrome), reduced intestinal absorption (e.g., malabsorptive disease, phosphate binders, dietary deficiency), reduced renal reabsorption (i.e., primary hyperparathyroidism, tubular disorders, eclampsia) or laboratory error (Allen-Durrance, 2017; DiBartola and Willard, 2012b). See Box 7iii.1 for a summary.

7iii.5 Supplementation of Calcium and Phosphorus

Several scenarios may exist where emergent administration of calcium is necessary to avoid life-threatening sequelae. In each clinical scenario it is prudent to consider the goal of the calcium administration, as this will dictate dose and rate of administration. Calcium is generally administered slowly, as a continuous rate infusion (CRI) with ECG monitoring to observe for any adverse drug reactions (e.g., bradycardia,

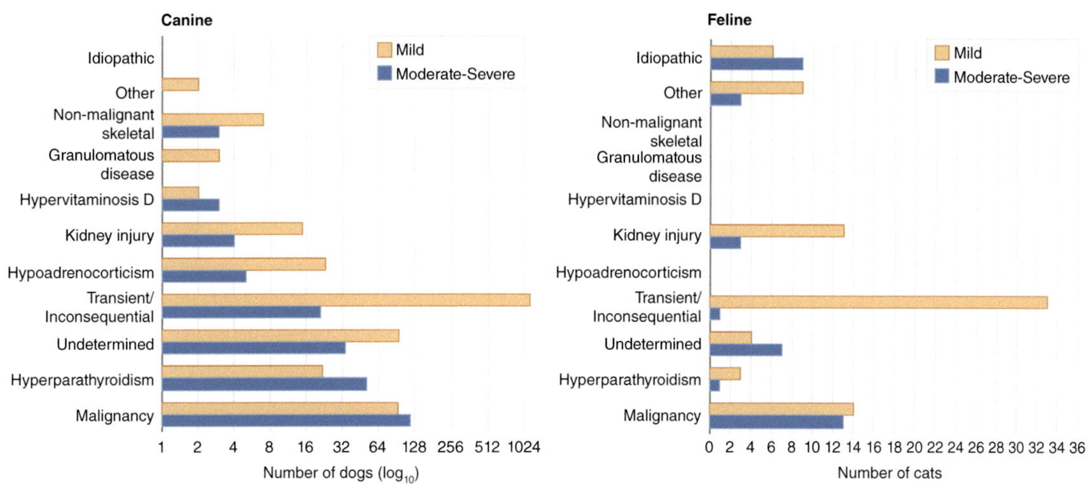

Fig. 7iii.2. Etiology of hypercalcemia as it correlates to severity in dogs and cats. (© The Ohio State University.) Data from Coady *et al.*, 2019.

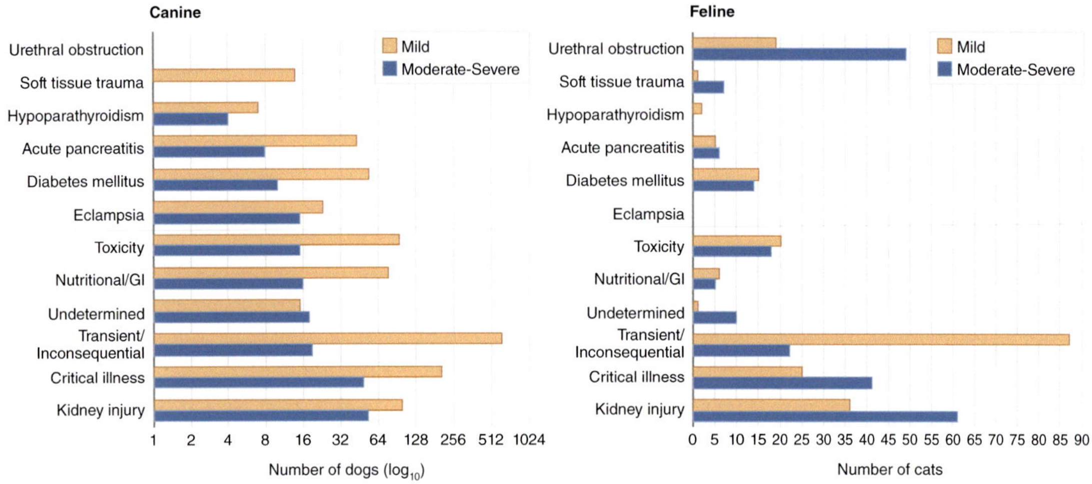

Fig. 7iii.3. Etiology of hypocalcemia as it correlates to severity in dogs and cats. (© The Ohio State University.) Data from Coady *et al.*, 2019.

Box 7iii.1. Causes of hyperphosphatemia and hypophosphatemia.

Hyperphosphatemia	Hypophosphatemia
Decreased excretion	**Cellular translocation**
Acute or chronic kidney disease	Insulin therapy
Cellular translocation	Respiratory alkalosis
Tumor lysis syndrome	Refeeding syndrome
Trauma	**Decreased intestinal absorption**
Metabolic acidosis	Malabsorptive disease
Increased absorption	Phosphate binders
Phosphate enema	**Decreased renal absorption**
Vitamin D toxicosis	Primary hyperparathyroidism
Growth	Tubular transport disorders
Laboratory error	

shortened QT interval). However, aggressive treatment in the form of a slow IV bolus (over 5–30 min) may be indicated for patients with severe clinical signs (such as malignant arrhythmias secondary to hyperkalemia or myoclonic disorders/seizures secondary to acute/severe hypocalcemia) (DiBartola and Willard, 2012a,b; Long *et al.*, 2018). In such clinical scenarios, the goal of treatment is to narrowly raise calcium levels enough to attenuate clinical signs. Attempts to normalize serum ionized calcium levels may lead to inadvertent consequences, including accidental hypercalcemia and hypercalciuria (DiBartola and Willard, 2012a). Once severe clinical signs are controlled, if the patient is expected to require continued calcium supplementation, a CRI is recommended (Table 7iii.1).

Similarly, hypophosphatemia may pose a significant threat to a patient, especially if reductions in serum phosphorus levels occur rapidly. Most notably, hemolysis may occur when levels fall below 1 mg/dl (<0.32 mmol/l) and neuromuscular signs can be seen that range from weakness to encephalopathic-like syndromes. Other consequences of hypophosphatemia may include impaired oxygen delivery, impaired leukocyte function, impaired platelet function, ileus, impaired cardiac contractility, and acid–base disturbances. Hypophosphatemia may be mild (2–2.5 mg/dl, 0.65–0.81 mmol/l), moderate (1–1.9 mg/dl, 0.32–0.61 mmol/l) or severe (<1 mg/dl, <0.32 mmol/l). Patients with moderate hypophosphatemia that are at risk for further reductions in phosphorus levels (e.g., DKA patient receiving insulin therapy) and any critically ill patient in the severe category generally require parenteral supplementation (Felsenfeld and Levine, 2012; Allen-Durrance, 2017; Thomovsky, 2017). In patients with renal insufficiency, phosphate replacement should be reduced by at least 50%. Additionally, phosphate therapy can exacerbate existing hypocalcemia. Conversely, phosphate therapy in the face of hypercalcemia can lead to calcium–phosphate precipitation, soft tissue mineralization and acute kidney injury (Felsenfeld and Levine, 2012). Given the relationship between these two, aberrancies in calcium levels warrant caution when considering phosphorus supplementation. They should also never be administered through the same infusion line. See Table 7iii.2 for dosing information.

Table 7iii.1. Parenteral calcium solutions and dosing information. Data from DiBartola and Willard (2012a).

Drug	Calcium content	Dose	Indication	Adverse event monitoring	Comment
Calcium gluconate 10% solution	9.3 mg Ca/ml[a] 90.7 mg gluconate/ml	Bolus: 0.5–1.5 ml/kg IV to effect CRI: 2–15 mg/kg/h	ECG changes secondary to hyperkalemia (absent P waves, widened QRS complex, tented T waves): administer dose over 5–10 min Acute management of clinical hypocalcemia (fasciculations/ tremors, tetany, seizures): administer dose over 20–30 min	Discontinue if bradycardia observed or shortened QT interval. For $CaCl_2$ 10% formula: extremely caustic if injected perivascular; ensure IV catheter integrity or use central line access	For treatment of hyper[K]: onset of action for either formula is <3 min with duration of action 20–60 min, repeat dose in 5 min if no improvement in ECG is seen
Calcium chloride 10% solution	27.2 mg Ca/ml 72.8 mg chloride/ml	Bolus: 5–15 mg/kg IV to effect CRI: 2–15 mg/kg/h			

[a]While this is a 10% solution, there are only 9.3 mg/mL of elemental calcium and 90.7 mg/mL of gluconate (total 100 mg/mL). Dosing is based on elemental calcium for the CRI. AV, atrioventricular; CRI, continuous rate infusion; IV, intravenous.

Notes:

- Do not mix calcium solutions with bicarbonate-containing fluids, because precipitation may occur.
- Not recommended to give calcium salts subcutaneously, even if diluted, due to risk of local necrosis and abscess formation.
- There is no difference in effectiveness of intravenous calcium salts when the dose is based on elemental calcium content.

Table 7iii.2. Parenteral phosphate solutions and dosing information. Data from DiBartola and Willard (2012b).

Solution	pH	Osmolality (mOsm/kg)	Phosphate (mmol/ml)	Potassium (meq/ml)	Sodium (meq/ml)	Dose	Indication	Adverse event monitoring
Potassium phosphate (K_2HPO_4)	6.6	5840	3	4.4	0	0.01–0.06 mmol/ kg/h Diluted in 0.9% saline	Phosphorus < 1mg/dl (0.32 mmol/l) Phosphorus 1–1.9 mg/dl (0.32–0.61 mmol/l) with concurrent insulin CRI Clinical signs attributed to hypophosphatemia	Over-supplementation can lead to hypocalcemia, soft tissue calcification, acute kidney injury and hyperphosphatemia Reassess phosphorus levels every 4–8 h
Sodium phosphate (Na_2HPO_4)	5.7	5580	3	0	4			

Clinical Case 7iii.1: Hyperkalemia

A 6-year-old male neutered strictly indoor domestic shorthair cat weighing 5.6 kg presents with a history of vomiting and becoming progressively lethargic over the past 24 h. The patient is examined to be approximately 6% dehydrated with a heart rate of 140 bpm and a painful firm distended bladder. The patient is diagnosed with circulatory shock and a urethral obstruction. The diagnostics provided in the table below and Fig. 7iii.4 were obtained at presentation.

Parameter	Value	S.I. (US)	Reference low	Reference high
pH	7.186		7.265	7.424
Na	140 (140)	mmol/l (mEq/l)	146.2 (146.2)	156.2 (156.2)
K	8.1 (8.1)	mmol/l (mEq/l)	3.42 (3.42)	4.71 (4.71)
iCa	1.02 (4.10)	mmol/l (mg/dl)	1.17 (4.7)	1.35 (5.4)
HCT	44.0 (44.0)	%	36 (36)	50 (50)
Cl	111.2 (11.2)	mmol/l (mEq/l)	117 (117)	125 (125)
Glucose	265.00	mmol/l (mg/dl)	3.99 (72)	7.32 (132)
Lactate	3.50	mmol/l (mg/dl)	1.1 (9.9)	3.5 (31.5)
iMg	1.2000	mmol/l (mg/dl)	0.33 (0.80)	0.49 (1.19)
BE-ecf	−13.3 (−13.3)	mmol/l (mEq/l)	−5.6 (−5.6)	0.8 (0.8)
HCO_3	15.2 (15.2)	mmol/l (mEq/l)	17.6 (17.6)	22.2 (22.2)
Gap	20.70	mmol/l (mEq/l)	12 (12)	20 (20)
BUN	>36 (>100)	mmol/l (mg/dl)	7.85 (22)	11.8 (33)
Creatinine	594.8 (7.8)	µmol/l (mg/dl)	53.4 (0.7)	144.9 (1.9)

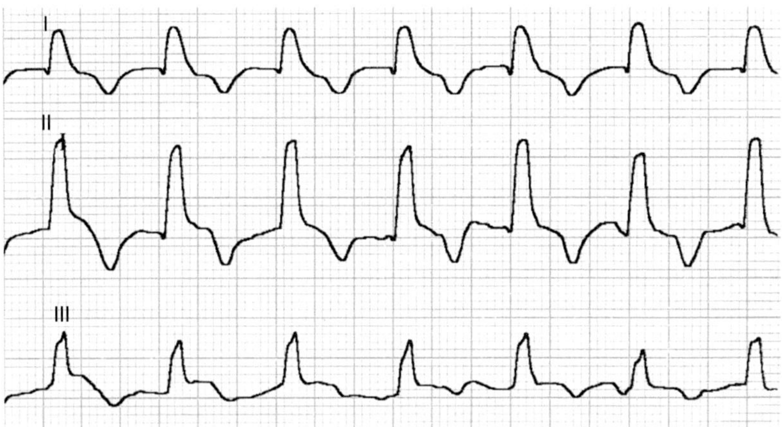

Fig. 7iii.4. Feline ECG tracing demonstrating atrial standstill and intraventricular conduction delay consistent with a sinoventricular rhythm secondary to hyperkalemia. (Image courtesy of Dr Karsten Schober, The Ohio State University Veterinary Medical Center: Cardiology and Interventional Medicine Department. Image last modified 24 March 2021.)

The patient's circulatory shock and marked hyperkalemia were addressed with a crystalloid bolus at 5 ml/kg administered over 20 min to encourage circulating volume and dilute serum potassium levels. Methadone at 0.2 mg/kg was administered for pain. The absent P waves and widened QRS complex were addressed with calcium gluconate 10% solution for cardiomyocyte membrane stabilization. The following calculation was used:

Continued

Clinical Case 7iii.1: Continued.

Calcium gluconate 10% emergency dosing:
1 ml/kg × 5.6 kg = 5.6 ml over 5 min

ECG monitoring was continuous. The ECG normalized 5 min after administration and the heart rate improved to 160 bpm. The patient was subsequently sedated with midazolam at 0.2 mg/kg and alfaxalone at 0.5 mg/kg as needed to effect for the unblocking procedure. The ECG was monitored for the duration of the procedure. The unblocking procedure was completed in 10 min; additional doses of calcium gluconate were not necessary in this case. The patient was monitored with telemetry for 6–8 h as ongoing fluid therapy was provided and urine output was monitored; recovery was considered to be uneventful.

Clinical Case 7iii.2: Periparturient hypocalcemia

A 4-year-old female intact Yorkshire Terrier mix presents 6 days post-partum for a 12 h history of restlessness, trembling, diarrhea and a possible seizure. On initial assessment the patient is found to be in a thin body condition (weight 3.9 kg) with developed mammary chains. The patient was anxious, panting, and exhibiting generalized muscle fasciculations and fine tremors. An elevated temperature of 104.2°F (40°C) and sinus tachycardia of 190 bpm were measured. The following blood work was obtained at the time of IV catheter placement:

Parameter	Value	S.I. (US)	Reference low	Reference high
pH	7.32		7.265	7.424
Na	152.7 (152.7)	mmol/l (mEq/l)	146.2 (146.2)	156.2 (156.2)
K	3.8 (3.8)	mmol/l (mEq/l)	3.42 (3.42)	4.71 (4.71)
iCa	0.72 (2.9)	mmol/l (mg/dl)	1.17 (4.7)	1.35 (5.4)
HCT	30 (30)	%	36 (36)	50 (50)
Cl	120.2 (120.2)	mmol/l (mEq/l)	117 (117)	125 (125)
Glucose	5.99 (108)	mmol/l (mg/dl)	3.99 (72)	7.32 (132)
Lactate	4.5 (40.5)	mmol/l (mg/dl)	1.1 (9.9)	3.5 (31.5)
iMg	0.33 (0.80)	mmol/l (mg/dl)	0.33 (0.80)	0.49 (1.19)
BE-ecf	–4.3 (–4.2)	mmol/l (mEq/l)	–5.6 (–5.6)	0.8 (0.8)
HCO_3	20.2 (20.2)	mmol/l (mEq/l)	17.6 (17.6)	22.2 (22.2)
Gap result	16.7 (16.7)	mmol/l (mEq/l)	12 (12)	20 (20)
BUN	13.6 (38.0)	mmol/l (mg/dl)	7.85 (22)	11.8 (33)
Creatinine	144.9 (1.9)	μmol/l (mg/dl)	53.4 (0.7)	144.9 (1.9)

A diagnosis of periparturient hypocalcemia was confirmed. Immediate treatment with calcium gluconate 10% was initiated at 10 mg/kg (1 ml/kg) IV over 20 min. Continuous ECG monitoring was employed for the duration of the infusion to observe for bradycardia or altered ECG morphology as this would warrant temporary infusion discontinuation and a slower subsequent rate (Davidson, 2012). Fifteen minutes following the initiation of the infusion the heart rate improved to 140 bpm, muscle fasciculation/trembling improved, and the body temperature was re-taken to be 103.0°F (39.4°C). An ionized calcium level was obtained following the 20 min infusion.

Parameter	Value	Unit	Reference low	Reference high
iCa	1.07 (4.3)	mmol/l (mg/dl)	1.17 (4.7)	1.35 (5.4)

Continued

Clinical Case 7iii.2: Continued.

A calcium gluconate CRI was then initiated using a syringe pump to maintain the patient in an asymptomatic state and provide ongoing calcium support until oral calcium supplementation (e.g. calcium carbonate) could be started. The CRI dose was chosen arbitrarily from the suggested range (2–15 mg/kg) with intent to adjust/discontinue based on subsequent calcium level monitoring, clinical signs, and the patient's oral intake. The following calculations were used for the CRI formulation.

1. Calcium gluconate continuous rate infusion dose:
   5 mg/kg × 3.9 kg = 20 mg/h
2. Calcium gluconate continuous rate infusion:
   20 mg/h ÷ 9.3 mg/ml elemental calcium = 2.2 ml/h CRI

Alternative methods for adding calcium gluconate to saline solutions can be employed. When using linear maintenance fluid rates for canines (60 ml/kg/day) and utilizing calcium gluconate 10% (9.3 mg elemental Ca/ml), elemental calcium supplementation rates of 1, 2 or 3 mg/kg/h are achieved by adding calcium gluconate 10% at 10, 20 or 30 ml, respectively, to a 250 ml bag of saline. Avoid crystalloids containing additives that can lead to calcium precipitation (e.g. lactate, acetate, bicarbonate or phosphate)

Note: In resource-limited settings, a controversial albeit alternative option is to administer calcium gluconate (not calcium chloride) at 0.5–1.5 ml/kg diluted 1:2 with normal saline via a subcutaneous route. This dosing is repeated every 6–8 h until the patient stabilizes and oral supplementation can be started. Subcutaneous calcium gluconate should always be diluted and divided between several sites if giving more than 5 ml, due to risk of local site irritation (Davidson, 2012). Caution should be exercised, as subcutaneous administration can cause pain, irritation, necrosis, abscessation or granuloma formation. As such, these methods have largely fallen out of favor and are no longer recommended as safe (Serrano and McMillan, 2009; DiBartola and Willard, 2012a).

Oral supplementation with calcium is often necessary for ongoing management of clinical hypocalcemic periparturient patients; doses of elemental calcium at 10–30 mg/kg q8h or 25–50 mg/kg/day have been published (Davidson, 2012; de Brito Galvão *et al.*, 2017b; Gonzales, 2018). Calcium carbonate in the form of 500 mg tablets purchased over the counter most commonly contains 200 mg of elemental calcium (Davidson, 2012; Gonzales, 2018).

Clinical Case 7iii.3: Phosphorus supplementation in diabetic ketoacidosis

A 10-year-old female spayed Pug weighing 9.8 kg presents for a 48 h history of hyporexia and two episodes of vomiting. The patient is a known diabetic and receives 11 units of porcine zinc insulin every 12 h with reportedly moderate control. On physical examination the patient has advanced cataracts, marked abdominal pain and is approximately 7% clinically dehydrated. An abdominal ultrasound is performed and is most consistent with pancreatitis and enteritis. The following diagnostics were obtained at presentation:

Parameter	Value	S.I. (US)	Reference low	Reference high
HCT	62 (62)	%	40 (40)	59 (59)
Plasma protein	81 (8.1)	g/l (g/dl)	56 (5.6)	73 (7.3)
BUN	10.7 (30)	mmol/l (mg/dl)	3.57 (10)	9.64 (27)
Creatinine	45.75 (0.60)	µmol/l (mg/dl)	7.63 (0.1)	99.1 (1.3)
Phosphorus	0.45 (1.4)	mmol/l (mg/dl)	0.71 (2.2)	2.03 (6.3)
Calcium – total	2.15 (8.6)	mmol/l (mg/dl)	2.27 (9.1)	2.88 (11.5)
Sodium	151 (151)	mmol/l (mEq/l)	145 (145)	154 (154)
Potassium	3.4 (3.4)	mmol/l (mEq/l)	3.9 (3.9)	5.5 (5.5)
Chloride	113 (113)	mmol/l (mEq/l)	107 (107)	(118) 118
Anion Gap	16 (16)	mmol/l (mEq/l)	15 (15)	25 (25)
Osmolality (calc)	309 (309)	mmol/kg (mOsm/kg)	289 (289)	308 (308)

Continued

Clinical Case 7iii.3: Continued.

Parameter	Value	S.I. (US)	Reference low	Reference high
Bicarbonate - total	15.1 (15.1)	mmol/l (mEq/l)	18 (18)	27 (27)
ALT – alanine amino transferase	1.82 (109)	µkat/l (IU/l)	0.3 (18)	1.8 (108)
AST – aspartate amino transferase	1.2 (72)	µkat/l (IU/l)	0.27 (16)	0.85 (51)
AP – alkaline phosphatase	2.37 (142)	µkat/l (IU/l)	0.2 (12)	2.22 (133)
CK – creatine kinase	2.24 (134)	µkat/l (IU/l)	0.89 (53)	(6.21) 372
Cholesterol	3.91 (151)	mmol/l (mg/dl)	3.16 (122)	8.94 (345)
Bilirubin - total	5.47 (0.32)	µmol/l (mg/dl)	0.86 (0.05)	3.42 (0.2)
Total protein - serum	81 (8.1)	g/l (g/dl)	51 (5.1)	71 (7.1)
Albumin	3.3 (0.33)	g/l (g/dl)	3.3 (0.33)	4.2 (0.42)
Globulin	18 (1.80)	g/l (g/dl)	17 (1.7)	34 (3.4)
A/G ratio	18.3 (1.83)	g/l (g/dl)	0 (0)	0 (0)
Glucose - serum	25.2 (454)	mmol/l (mg/dl)	3.72 (67)	7.05 (127)
GGT	.08 (5)	µkat/l (IU/l)	0 (0)	0.37 (22.3)
Ketones (Point of Care Analyzer)	3.8	mmol/l	0	0.32

The patient was diagnosed with diabetic ketoacidosis, mild hypokalemia, and moderate hypophosphatemia. A rehydration plan with appropriate electrolyte supplementation was initiated for 4 h prior to starting intravenous insulin therapy.

Note: When simultaneous supplementation of phosphorus and potassium are needed, two approaches can be employed assuming that supplementation of phosphorus is with potassium phosphate (potassium 4.4 meEq/ml, phosphorus 3 mmol/ml), and supplementation of potassium is with potassium chloride (potassium 2 mEq/ml). Published dosages for phosphorus supplementation are 0.01–0.06 mmol/kg/h (DiBartola and Willard, 2012b) and 0.01–0.2 mmol/kg/h (Drobatz *et al.*, 2019). It is recommended that supplementation rates of potassium do not exceed 0.5 mEq/kg/h due to risk of cardiac arrhythmia (DiBartola and Willard, 2012b; Drobatz et al., 2019).

1. The first approach involves selecting a phosphorus supplementation dose in mmol/kg/h, then calculating how much potassium in mEq/kg/h will be supplemented with that rate. The potassium being provided through the KPhos is then subtracted from the total desired KCl dose.

2. The second approach involves selecting a desired potassium supplementation rate. This rate is then divided 25%–75% or 50%–50% between KPhos and KCl, respectively. With this approach, the KPhos (potassium 4.4 mEq/ml) and the KCl (potassium 2 mEq/ml) are dosed based on potassium concentrations. This often provides an adequate amount of PO_4 while guaranteeing potassium dosing goals.

The following calculations were used to calculate a rehydration fluid therapy plan (see Chapter 6ii for more information), phosphorus supplementation, and potassium supplementation; electrolytes were added to a 1 l bag of isotonic crystalloids.

1. Maintenance fluid rate (based on allometric scale): $9.8\ kg^{0.75} \times 132 = 731$ ml/day ÷ 14 h/day = 30 ml/h
2. 7% rehydration fluid rate (replaced over 12 h): 0.07 × 9.8 kg = 0.686 l deficit × 1000 ml/l ÷ 12 h = 57 ml/h
3. Total fluid rate: 30 ml/h + 57 ml/h = 87 ml/h of calcium-free balanced crystalloid
4. Phosphorus supplementation rate (KPhos): (0.03 mmol/kg/h) × 9.8 kg = (0.3 mmol/h) ÷ (3 mmol Ph/ml KPhos) = 0.1 ml/h KPhos
5. Potassium achieved with KPhos: (0.1 ml/h KPhos) × 4.4 (mEq K /ml KPhos) = 0.44 mEq/h K from KPhos
6. Total desired potassium supplementation rate: 0.3 mEq/kg/h × 9.8 kg = 3 mEq/h K
7. required from KCl: (3 mEq/h K) – (0.44 mEq/h K) = (2.6 mEq/h from KCl) ÷ (2 mEqK / ml KCl) = 1.3 ml/h KCl
8. Totals to add to 1 l calcium-free balanced crystalloid:
   1000 ml ÷ 87 ml/h = 11.5 h lifespan of 1 l
   0.1 ml/h × 11.5 h = 1.15 ml KPhos added to 1 l
   1.3 ml/h × 11.5 h = 15 ml KCl added to 1 l

The calculations for the alternative method of supplementation are as follows:

Continued

Clinical Case 7iii.3: Continued.

1. Total desired potassium supplementation rate: 0.3 mEq/kg/h × 9.8 kg = 3 mEq/h K
2. 25% potassium as KPhos (potassium 4.4 mEq/ml): 0.25 × 3 mEq/h = 0.75 mEq/h ÷ 4.36 mEq/ml = 0.17 ml/h KPhos
3. 75% potassium as KCl (potassium 2 mEq/ml): 0.75 × 3 mEq/h = 2.25 mEq/h – 2 mEq/ml – 1.1 ml/h KCl
4. Totals to add to 1 l calcium-free balanced crystalloid: 1000 ml – 87 ml/h = 11.5 h lifespan of 1 l

The alternative method provides KPhos at 0.17 ml/h which equates to phosphorus supplementation at 0.05 mmol/kg/h, which is at the higher end of the dosing interval. As such, frequent monitoring of phosporus levels is indicated so as not to cause inadvertent harm of over-supplementation.

References

Allen-Durrance, A.E. (2017) A quick reference on phosphorus. *Veterinary Clinics of North America Small Animal Practice* 47, 257–262.

Bergwitz, C. and Juppner, H. (2010). Regulation of phosphate homeostasis by PTH, vitamin D, and FGF23. *Annual Review of Medicine* 61, 91–104.

Coady, M., Fletcher, D.J. and Goggs, R. (2019). Severity of ionized hypercalcemia and hypocalcemia is associated with etiology in dogs and cats. *Frontiers in Veterinary Science* 6, 276.

Davidson, A.P. (2012). Reproductive causes of hypocalcemia. *Topics in Companion Animal Medicine* 27, 165-6.

de Brito Galvão, J.F., Schenk, P.A. and Chew, D.J. (2017a) A quick reference on hypercalcemia. *Veterinary Clinics of North America Small Animal Practice* 47, 241–248.

de Brito Galvão, J.F., Schenk, P.A. and Chew, D.J. (2017b) A quick reference on hypocalcemia. *Veterinary Clinics of North America Small Animal Practice* 47, 249–256.

DiBartola, S.P. and Willard, M.D. (2012a) Disorders of calcium: hypercalcemia and hypocalcemia. In: DiBartola, S.P. (ed.) *Fluid, Electrolyte, and Acid-Base Disorders in Small Animal Practice*, 4th edn. Elsevier Saunders, St Louis, Missouri, p. 175.

DiBartola, S.P. and Willard, M.D. (2012b) Disorders of phosphorus: hypophosphatemia and hyperphosphatemia. In: DiBartola, S.P (ed.) *Fluid, Electrolyte, and Acid-Base Disorders in Small Animal Practice*, 4th edn. Elsevier Saunders, St Louis, Missouri, p. 202.

Dittmer, K.E., Perera, K.C. and Elder, P.A. (2017) Serum fibroblast growth factor 23 concentrations in dogs with chronic kidney disease. *Research in Veterinary Science* 114, 348–350.

Drobatz, K.J., Hopper, K., Rozanski, E.A. and Silverstein, D.C. (eds) (2019) *Textbook of Small Animal Emergency Medicine*. John Wiley and Sons, Hoboken, New Jersey.

Erben, R.G. (2018) Physiological actions of fibroblast growth factor-23. *Frontiers in Endocrinology (Lausanne)* 9, 267.

Felsenfeld, A.J. and Levine, B.S. (2012) Approach to treatment of hypophosphatemia. *American Journal of Kidney Disease* 60, 655–661.

Gonzales, K. (2018) Periparturient diseases in the dam. *Veterinary Clinics of North America Small Animal Practice* 48, 663–681.

Huang, X., Jiang, Y. and Xia, W. (2013) FGF23 and phosphate wasting disorders. *Bone Research* 1, 120–132.

Long, B., Warix, J.R. and Koyfman, A. (2018) Controversies in management of hyperkalemia. *Journal of Emergency Medicine* 55, 192–205.

Molina, P.E. (2018). Parathyroid gland and Ca^{2+} and PO_4^- regulation. In: Molina, P.E. (ed.) *Endocrine Physiology*, 5th edn. McGraw Hill, New York, pp. 101–130.

Serrano, S. and McMillan, M. (2009) Dystocia. *Standards of Care: Emergency and Critical Care Medicine* 11, 1–5.

Thomovsky, E. (2017) Fluid and electrolyte therapy in diabetic ketoacidosis. *Veterinary Clinics of North America Small Animal Practice* 47, 491–503.

7iv Magnesium Supplementation

Julien Guillaumin

Colorado State University, Fort Collins, Colorado, USA

Magnesium is the fourth most abundant cation in the body and the second in the intracellular fluid compartment (Martin and Allen-Durrance, 2009). Distribution of magnesium across body compartments in veterinary species has not been well studied. In humans, almost the entire amount of total magnesium (99%) is located in intracellular stores. Bone storage accounts for two-thirds of magnesium, while 20% is found in muscles and 13% is found in other soft tissues. Only 1% of total magnesium is present in the extracellular fluid compartment and the approximate percentages of repartition within the extracellular fluid compartment are as follows (although variations of those percentages are found in the literature): 65% is ionized, 30% bound to proteins, and 5% in anion complexes (phosphates and sulphates) (Bateman, 2006). Magnesium concentrations are very tightly controlled within the body.

In some circumstances, the inability to measure ionized magnesium (which is the biologically active form) or interpret the meaning of total serum magnesium makes the diagnosis of magnesium disorders challenging. Also, magnesium concentrations can be reported in different units, which can also be confusing (Table 7iv.1). A magnesium level of 0.1 mmol/l equates to 0.24 mg/dl, so to convert mmol/l to mg/dl, multiply by 2.4. As magnesium is a divalent cation, 1 mmol/l is 2 mEq/l.

7iv.1 Physiological Role

While it is not given as much consideration as some of the other electrolytes, magnesium plays a very important role in numerous cellular metabolic processes. It is a co-factor for more than 300 enzymatic reactions within cells, such as phosphorylative oxidation, the Krebs cycle, protein synthesis, and most phosphate transfer reactions. Specifically, it is a coenzyme for Na-K-ATPase. Every molecule of ATP must be associated with a molecule of magnesium in order to be active (Elin, 1994). Through its effects on adenylate cyclase, a second messengers formation, and calcium ATPase, magnesium is also a signaling molecule in neurotransmission and has an important role in maintenance of the resting membrane potential in excitatory cells. Its role in the maintenance of neuromuscular function, including cardiac conduction and vascular smooth muscle tone, cannot be overestimated.

Magnesium is initially absorbed through the GI tract (particularly the ileum) through dietary intake, though the kidneys are primarily responsible for overall regulation of body magnesium levels. Unlike many electrolytes, which are primarily reabsorbed in the proximal tubule, 50–60% of magnesium is reabsorbed in the thick ascending loop of Henle (Bateman, 2006).

7iv.2 Clinical Signs

Severe clinical hypomagnesemia is rare in small animal medicine, and it is more common in food animals (e.g., grass tetany). However, the list of causes for hypomagnesemia include decreased dietary intake or increased losses through the kidneys or gastrointestinal tract. Hypomagnesia is also present in 20–65% of human ICU patients and it is associated with worse outcome (Dubé and Granry, 2003). In veterinary medicine, it has been shown that 54% of critically ill dogs and 23% of critically ill cats are hypomagnesemic (Cortes and Moses, 2007). Many syndromes that affect critically ill patients, including gastrointestinal disorders (e.g., diarrhea, vomiting), renal loss (e.g., osmotic diuresis, metabolic acidosis, kidney disease), and drug administration, can lead to hypomagnesemia (Box 7iv.1).

Clinical signs primarily relate to magnesium's role in neuromuscular function and cardiac conduction. The patient may exhibit non-specific signs of weakness or twitching, or may have dysphagia or dyspnea. In humans, various arrhythmias are associated

DOI: 10.1079/9781789243406.0074

with hypomagnesemia, including atrial fibrillation, supraventricular tachycardia, ventricular premature contractions, ventricular tachycardia, ventricular fibrillation, and torsade de pointes (Fig. 7iv.1). Severe hypomagnesemia may result in seizures, but neurological signs in small animal patients are uncommon (Bateman, 2006).

In addition to the cardiovascular and neurological effects, magnesium also plays an important role in renal potassium reabsorption. As previously mentioned, magnesium serves as a co-factor for the activity of the Na–K ATPase pump. As this pump helps to move potassium into the intracellular space, without magnesium there is an extracellular accumulation. Extracellular potassium will be filtered through the glomerulus, and with decreased magnesium (and thereby Na–K ATPase function) there will be reduced reabsorption. The result is a significant loss of potassium and the development or exacerbation of hypokalemia that is refractory to supplementation. Further compounding this is the fact that hypokalemia also promotes magnesium loss through the kidneys. In these circumstances it is essential to supplement both electrolytes.

Table 7iv.1. Normal magnesium (Mg) levels in companion animals.

	mmol/l	mg/dl	mEq/l
Total Mg (dog)	0.7–1.0	1.6–2.5	1.4–2.0
Ionized Mg (dog)	0.43–0.6		
Total Mg (cat)	0.8–1.0	1.9–2.6	1.6–2.0
Ionized Mg (cat)	0.43–0.7		

Box 7iv.1. Select causes of hypomagnesemia.

Decreased dietary intake

- Gastrointestinal
- Chronic diarrhea
- Malabsorptive syndromes
- Short bowel syndrome
- Inherited

Renal

- Diabetes mellitus/ketoacidosis
- Diuretics (furosemide)
- Osmotic agents
- Polyuric renal failure
- Fluid therapy/diuresis
- Hypokalemia/hypophosphatemia

7iv.3 Treatment

Clinical hypomagnesemia typically requires a total magnesium value of 0.2–0.5 mEq/l (0.3–0.6 mg/dl) but may also be asymptomatic. Both hypocalcemia and hypokalemia can be secondary to hypomagnesemia.

Treatment of hypomagnesemia in the critically ill and clinically affected patient will usually be accomplished with intravenous infusions. This may come in the form of emergency treatment (as might be needed for ventricular arrhythmias) and more chronic supplementation.

It is very important to avoid mistakes in administration and timing, as vial concentration and administration dose (i.e., per hour, per day) vary. Magnesium sulfate ($MgSO_4$) is the most commonly used supplementation and comes as a 10% solution, which contains magnesium at 0.8 mEq/ml, but can also come as a 50% solution, containing 4 mEq/ml (or 2 mmol/ml) (Fig. 7iv.2). If using the

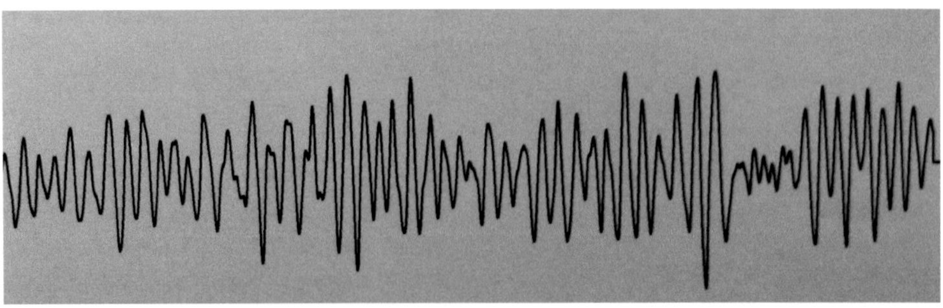

Fig. 7iv.1. Ventricular fibrillation torsade de pointes is a classic indication for emergency treatment with intravenous magnesium.

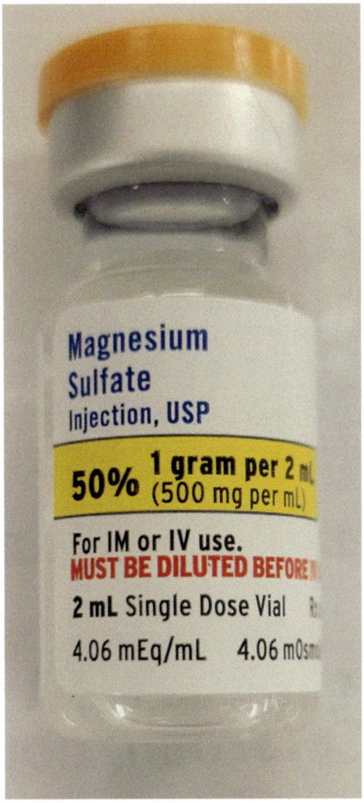

Fig. 7iv.2. Example of magnesium sulfate 50%, which contains magnesium at 4 mEq/ml (500 mg/ml).

50% solution it should be diluted to 20% or less. If the patient is concurrently hypocalcemic, magnesium chloride ($MgCl_2$) should be used instead of $MgSO_4$ since the sulfate ion will chelate calcium. Dilution of any magnesium sources should always be in 0.9% NaCl or 5% dextrose in water, avoiding any solutions that contain calcium or bicarbonate, as these may precipitate. Magnesium chloride ($MgCl_2$) can be supplied as a 20% solution, which contains magnesium at 1.98 mEq/ml (200 mg/ml).

Dose recommendations for emergency treatment, such as management of ventricular arrhythmias, is 0.15–0.3 mEq/kg (or 20–40 mg/kg) for $MgSO_4$ or $MgCl_2$, which can be given over 20–30 min (Bateman, 2006). This is a total dose/kg. Dose recommendation

Box 7iv.2. Dosing recommendations for magnesium supplementation.

Emergency/loading dose (over 20–30 min)

- $MgSO_4$ 0.15–0.3 mEq/kg (20–40 mg/kg)
- $MgCl_2$ 0.15–0.3 mEq/kg (15–30 mg/kg)

Constant rate infusion

- $MgSO_4$ 0.03–0.04 mEq/kg/h (3.5–5 mg/kg/h)
- $MgCl_2$ 0.03–0.04 mEq/kg/h (3–4.6 mg/kg/h)

Clinical Case 7iv.1

You have a 5 kg feline patient recently diagnosed with diabetic ketoacidosis (the same one from Chapter 7ii). Six hours ago she was started on a potassium CRI at 0.2 mEq/kg/h because her potassium was 3.1 mEq/l. You recheck her potassium and discover that it is now 2.8 mEq/l. You are not able to measure magnesium in your clinic, but the fact that her potassium has dropped despite supplementation has you worried that she has developed a clinically relevant deficiency. You decide to start supplementation at 0.04 mEq/kg/h (5 mg/kg/h) and have the 50% solution (4 mEq/ml or 500 mg/ml) on hand.

The first step is to dilute to 2% (0.16 mEq/ml or 20 mg/ml), as this solution is too hyperosmolar. You decide to make up 50 ml of stock solution:

V1 = (C2 × V2)/C1 = (2% × 50 ml)/50% = 2 ml of 50% $MgSO_4$ added to 48 ml of 0.9% NaCl = 0.16 mEq/ml $MgSO_4$

So, you plan to set your syringe pump to 0.04 mEq/kg/h, weight 5 kg, and concentration 0.16 mEq/l. This should yield a rate of:

0.04 mEq/kg/h × 5 kg ÷ 0.16 mEq/ml = 1.25 ml/h.

Alternatively, if a syringe pump is not available, you would need to add it to the patient's fluids (which is Plasma-Lyte running at 20 ml/h). You decide to use a buretrol to make up 120 ml at a time. Here is how you determine the volume of 50% $MgSO_4$ to add (ignoring the Mg already in the Plasma-Lyte):

Desired rate of infusion is 0.04 mEq/kg/h × 5 kg = 0.2 mEq/h

With a volume of 120 ml and a rate of 20 ml/h, there is 6 h of infusion in the buretrol

Total $MgSO_4$ needed = 0.2 mEq/h × 6 h = 1.2 mEq

Volume of $MgSO_4$ to add = 1.2 mEq ÷ 4 mEq/ml = 0.3 ml

Adding 0.3 ml of 50% $MgSO_4$ to 120 ml of Plasma-Lyte at 20 ml/h will deliver 0.04 mEq/kg/h.

for constant rate infusion (CRI) is 0.5–1 mEq/kg/day (0.25–1 mmol/kg/day). This is a *daily* dose/kg. When setting up as a CRI it may also be useful to set dosing per hour (0.03–0.04 mEq/kg/h or 3–5 mg/kg/h). See also Box 7iv.2 for dosing recommendations. Some isotonic fluids that contain magnesium (e.g., Plasma-Lyte) would provide magnesium at 0.15 mEq/kg/day if given at a maintenance rate. Hypermagnesemia related to over-supplementation is extremely rare as long as the infusion is set up appropriately and normal kidney function is present.

References

Bateman, S.W. (2006) Disorders of magnesium: magnesium deficit and excess. In: DiBartola, S.P. (ed.) *Fluid, Electrolyte, and Acid-Base Disorders in Small Animal Practice*. Saunders Elsevier, St Louis, Missouri, pp. 210–226.

Cortes, Y. and Moses, L. (2007) Magnesium disturbances in critically ill patients. *Compendium of Continuing Education for the Practicing Veterinarian* 29(7), 420–427.

Dubé, L. and Granry, J.C. (2003) The therapeutic use of magnesium in anesthesiology, intensive care and emergency medicine: a review. *Canadian Journal of Anesthesia* 50(7), 732–746.

Elin, R. (1994) Magnesium: the fifth but forgotten electrolyte. *American Journal of Clinical Pathology* 102(5), 616–622.

Martin, L.G. and Allen-Durrance, A. (2009) Magnesium and phosphate disorders. In: Silverstein, D.C. and Hopper, K. (eds) *Small Animal Critical Care Medicine*. Saunders Elsevier, St Louis, Missouri, pp. 240–243.

8i Special Considerations for Patients Experiencing Hemorrhage/Trauma

EDWARD COOPER

The Ohio State University, Columbus, Ohio, USA

The previous chapters have been geared toward a more generalized approach to fluid therapy, with the goal of then allowing extrapolation to a specific patient needing fluid resuscitation. However, there can be some disease processes, clinical conditions, and patient populations that warrant specific additional consideration. What follows in this chapter are selected clinical circumstances and case examples for which fluid therapy may be more challenging, nuanced, or associated with an increased risk of complications. While certainly not meant to be exhaustive, the goal is to highlight those circumstances that are more commonly experienced in veterinary medicine and which might warrant special consideration. Please note that, below, there is a certain amount of repetition from Chapter 6i, to save the reader from frequent cross-referencing.

8i.1 Pathophysiology of Trauma/ Hemorrhage

Traumatic injury is a common reason for presentation to veterinary hospitals, particularly in the emergency setting. While the location and severity can vary greatly, these patients can experience several sequelae, including pain, stress, musculoskeletal injuries, traumatic brain injury, respiratory compromise, and hemorrhagic shock. As a result, many of these patients may benefit from fluids to help restore circulating volume and support tissue perfusion. However, the complex nature of trauma and hemorrhage, as well as additional considerations imposed by the site(s) of injury, can complicate fluid therapy in these patients. While an extensive review is beyond the scope of this chapter (for more information see Muir, 2006; Palmer, 2017; Cooper, 2019), some consideration of the pathophysiology associated with traumatic injury and hemorrhage helps to set the stage for optimizing the approach to fluid administration (see also Chapter 6i).

Significant hemorrhage can be a major contributor to morbidity and mortality in the trauma patient. As described in Chapter 6i, acute loss of circulating volume will be the largest contributor to the development of shock and eventual cardiovascular collapse (Table 8i.1). In addition, the loss of red blood cells will lead to progressive anemia and decreased oxygen-carrying capacity. Plasma proteins (like albumin and coagulation factors) will also be lost and promote the development of hypoproteinemia and impaired coagulation. In this regard it can become apparent that blood loss can promote further blood loss, at least until hemostasis is achieved or perfusing pressure gets low enough (as all bleeding stops eventually).

Tissue damage secondary to trauma will trigger stimulation of the sympathetic nervous system (SNS) and rapid activation of local and systemic inflammatory responses. The SNS will promote tachycardia and peripheral vasoconstriction in an effort to improve cardiac output and maintain perfusion pressure. At the same time the inflammatory system tends to promote vasodilation and increase vascular permeability. This phenomenon has been termed trauma-induced capillary leak syndrome and is related to disruption of the endothelial glycocalyx and cell junctions (Cotton *et al.*, 2006; Lenz *et al.*, 2007; Stein and Scalea, 2012). This leads to an increased tendency for fluid and protein to move from the vascular compartment into the interstitial space. The resulting decrease in circulating volume can then contribute to impaired tissue perfusion, lactate production, and development of metabolic acidosis. Interestingly, the combination of tissue injury and hemorrhage magnifies the

DOI: 10.1079/9781789243406.0081

Table 8i.1. Classification of acute hemorrhage based on % loss of circulating volume. (Modified from the American College of Surgeons Advanced Trauma Life Support manual for canine and feline patients.)

Parameter	Class I	Class II	Class III	Class IV
Blood loss (%)	<15%	15–30%	30–40%	>40%
Heart rate (beats/min)				
Dog	100–120	120–140	140–180	>180
Cat	180–200	200–220	>220	>220 or <160[a]
Mucous membranes	Pink	Pale pink	Pale	White
Capillary refill	<2 sec	2–3 sec	3–4 sec	>4 sec, undetectable
Pulse quality	↔	↓	↓↓	↓↓ to absent
Blood pressure	↔	↔ to ↓	↓	↓↓
Mentation	Normal	Quiet	Dull	Stupor to coma

[a] Reflects the potential for cats to become bradycardic in shock. ↔ reflects no expected change.

impact of either (Muir, 2006). Said another way, a bleeding trauma patient will have more rapid progression and increased mortality than a patient with non-traumatic hemorrhage (e.g., bleeding splenic mass) at a comparable level of blood loss (Rady, 1994).

In conjunction with activation of the inflammatory system, significant derangements related to coagulation can develop. **Acute traumatic coagulopathy** (ATC) is a complex process that results in hypocoagulability (decreased clot formation) and hyperfibrinolysis (enhanced clot breakdown). These changes, which can occur within the first hour after severe trauma, are thought to be the results of several factors (**Box 8i.1**) and can lead to exacerbation of hemorrhage (Palmer and Martin, 2014). Fluid resuscitative efforts can further add to these factors and worsen coagulopathy (part of a process referred to as trauma-induced coagulopathy).

Patients experiencing significant trauma can also develop hypothermia secondary to impaired perfusion and increased exposure (from open wounds). Administration of cold resuscitative fluids can serve to further decrease body temperature. Hypothermia can be deleterious, as it can lead to worsening of coagulopathy, decreased cardiac function, arrhythmias, and altered metabolism. Along similar lines, progressive acidosis from lactic accumulation or administration of high chloride-containing fluids (0.9% NaCl) will also affect coagulation, catecholamine function, and assorted other enzymatic functions. The combination of coagulopathy, hypothermia, and acidosis creates a vicious cycle often referred to as the "lethal triad" (Fig. 8i.1).

Given the potential for trauma and hemorrhage to progress (rapidly) through this life-threatening process, taking every opportunity to control bleeding, restore perfusion, and limit ongoing tissue injury is essential to successful management. Thoughtful fluid administration is thereby a key aspect of resuscitative efforts.

Box 8i.1. Factors that contribute to the development of ATC (from Palmer, 2017).

- Tissue injury
- Hypoperfusion
- Systemic inflammation
- Metabolic acidosis
- Hypothermia
- Hemodilution

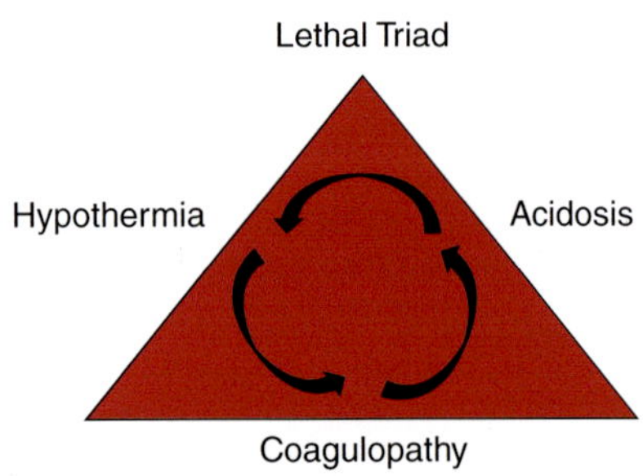

Fig. 8i.1. Schematic representation of the "lethal triad". Coagulopathy, hypothermia, and acidosis all contribute to clinical worsening in patients experiencing severe traumatic injury.

8i.2 What Type of Fluid?

Many of the general considerations regarding which fluid types might be optimally applied to patients experiencing trauma and/or hemorrhage have been

Table 8i.2. Recommended uses for various fluid types in trauma/hemorrhage.

Fluid type	Recommended use
Hypotonic crystalloid	Contraindicated
Balanced electrolyte solution	Reasonable initial fluid choice, but should be used judiciously
0.9% NaCl	Contraindicated
Hypertonic saline	Patients with traumatic brain injury Impending cardiovascular collapse Part of low-volume resuscitation strategy
Synthetic colloids	Contraindicated unless natural colloids unavailable
Natural colloids Blood products	Recommended for patients with moderate to severe hemorrhage

covered in Chapters 3, 4, and 6. Given the pathogenesis described above, the key factors to consider are increased vascular permeability, anemia, hypoproteinemia, coagulopathy, acidosis, and hypothermia. So, it becomes a function of determining which fluid types will best serve to address these issues (Table 8i.2).

As is always the case with resuscitation, use of **hypotonic** fluids is contraindicated. Relative to cost and availability, a balanced electrolyte solution is a reasonable starting fluid for the initial stages of resuscitation, and provision of maintenance requirements in ongoing fluid therapy. However, these fluids should be used judiciously, given the large volumes needed, and the potential to exacerbate tissue edema, hemodilution, and coagulopathy (Palmer, 2017; Hall and Drobatz, 2021). If possible, using warmed fluids (for example, kept in an incubator) will help to lessen the potential to worsen hypothermia. Use of 0.9% NaCl should be avoided as the high chloride content will contribute to acidosis and could be associated with increased risk of acute kidney injury (Semler and Kellum, 2019).

Hypertonic crystalloids, i.e., hypertonic saline (HTS) (e.g., 7% NaCl) have potential applications in these patients. Given the dual effect of expanding vascular volume and promoting osmotic reduction in intracranial pressure, perhaps the clearest indication for HTS is in patients with concurrent traumatic brain injury (TBI). In addition, the ability to expand the vascular volume with the administration of a relatively small amount is associated with less tissue edema and long-term hemodilution. However, the effect of HTS will be short-lived and will not result in a sustained volume expansion. For patients with active hemorrhage, it is also possible that the acute increase in perfusion pressure could serve to exacerbate bleeding. With these considerations in mind, aside from use with TBI, HTS is best used in circumstances of impending cardiovascular collapse to "buy time" while other fluids are administered.

As explained in Ch. 6i.2.4, synthetic colloids (such as VetStarch) hold some appeal, given the ability to increase circulating volume with less total administration compared with isotonic crystalloids (and so less tissue edema, hemodilution, etc.). In addition, they may be more readily available and cost effective compared with blood products. However, significant concerns have been raised regarding the potential for synthetic colloids to cause and/or contribute to coagulopathy and acute kidney injury. These considerations make their use in trauma/hemorrhaging patients much less ideal and should be avoided. That said, for patients not responding to crystalloids, limited use of synthetic colloids may be considered, especially when natural colloids/blood products are not available (Adamik and Yozova, 2021). Ongoing administration of synthetic colloids for oncotic support is not recommended.

For a number of reasons, natural colloids/blood products are the ideal fluid for patients experiencing moderate to severe hemorrhage. Blood products offer the ability to "replace that which has been lost", including red blood cells, coagulation factors, and plasma proteins (thus reducing tissue edema, hemodilution, coagulopathy, and hypoproteinemia). In this regard, **fresh whole blood** would be the optimal product to use (Hall and Drobatz, 2021). If not available, then split products of **packed red blood cells** and **fresh frozen plasma** (given at a 1:1 ratio) would be the next option and also provide significant benefit. **Autotransfusion** is also a consideration, as this gives the ability to return autologous red blood cells and some plasma proteins. It is important to note that autotransfused blood will have significantly reduced clotting factor concentrations (as coagulation is activated once blood has extravasated). Concurrent administration of plasma products should then be considered. Overall limitations for use of blood products include availability, cost, and the potential for transfusion reactions. In addition, rapid infusion of refrigerated/thawed blood products (e.g., massive transfusion protocols) could contribute to hypothermia and/or cause hypocalcemia from citrate chelation.

While certainly not a fluid type, another important consideration in the management of bleeding trauma patients is the use of an **antifibrinolytic agent** such as aminocaproic acid or tranexamic acid. As previously mentioned, ATC can be associated with hyperfibrinolysis, which can set the stage for excessive bleeding. These medications can decrease clot breakdown and have been shown to be beneficial in human trauma patients (Shakur *et al.*, 2010). There is less definitive evidence in the veterinary literature, and ideally the decision to use antifibrinolytics should be based on viscoelastic coagulation testing (such as thromboelastography) demonstrating hyperfibrinolysis (Hall and Drobatz, 2021). However, given the limited availability of these tests in veterinary medicine, it is reasonable to consider use of antifibrinolytics in bleeding trauma patients that are not responding to hemorrhage control and fluid resuscitation (Hall and Drobatz, 2021). Timing is also not entirely clear, but the optimal window is likely within 8 h of the traumatic event, when patients are more likely to be experiencing ATC. Beyond that, and certainly past 24 h, trauma patients are more likely to be hypercoagulable, making these medications contraindicated (Palmer and Martin, 2014).

8i.3 How Much/How Fast?

The question regarding how much fluid should be used and rate of administration in trauma and bleeding patients has received considerable attention and undergone significant revision. The "classic" approach (large volumes given quickly) had been the mainstay fluid resuscitation for decades, and was largely based on the notion that restoring circulating volume as quickly as possible is ideal. This approach was supported by early experimental hemorrhage models which suggested that for isotonic crystalloids it was necessary to administer three times the amount of blood lost in order to achieve resuscitation (the 3-to-1 rule) (Santry and Alam, 2010). With this, the classic resuscitation strategy could result in giving an entire circulating blood volume, or more (see Chapter 6i for more information).

However, more recently this approach has been called into question with the concern that large-volume rapid administration of fluids (particularly isotonic crystalloids) may have some adverse effects. This notion first came to the forefront in circumstances of the actively bleeding trauma patient. While initially it seems intuitive that the bleeding patient needs volume replaced rapidly, doing so with non-blood products (crystalloids, synthetic colloids) can result in edema, hemodilution, worsening coagulopathy, clot disruption, and exacerbation of hemorrhage (Dutton, 2007). See Chapter 6i for additional mechanisms of adverse effects. So, while there is transient improvement in blood pressure and clinical status, the patient declines from continued blood loss. This sets the stage for the "resuscitation rollercoaster", with ups and downs after each bolus and ultimately diminishing returns. In this regard, the benefits of a more cautious/restrictive approach to fluid therapy start to make sense for patients experiencing uncontrolled hemorrhage (Palmer, 2017), and with potential application to other circumstances of fluid resuscitation (such as sepsis, obstructive shock, and severe dehydration).

The goal of this more restrictive (revised) approach is that the volume of isotonic crystalloid is less, and the timeframe of administration is slower. As no specific guidelines have been established, a reasonable starting point for "less" is half the dose given in the classic approach (e.g., an isotonic crystalloid at 10–15 ml/kg rather than 20–30 ml/kg) administered over a similar or "slower" period of time (e.g., 20–30 min instead of 15–20 min). The result is a "slowless" rather than a bolus. The slowless can be given 1–2 times before deciding whether additional fluid administration is likely to be helpful (see Table 8i.3 and Fig. 8i.2 for additional recommendations).

Patients with moderate to severe hemorrhage, especially those that do not stabilize with limited crystalloid administration, will likely require the provision of blood products if available (fresh whole blood, or packed red blood cells and fresh frozen plasma in a 1:1 ratio). In these circumstances it is still preferred to titrate carefully, giving blood products as quickly as needed, but as slowly as will be tolerated. As an example, with catastrophic hemorrhage it may be necessary to perform a "**massive transfusion**", defined as the administration of more than a full circulating volume within 24 h, or half a circulating volume within 8 h (Patil and Shetmahajan, 2014). With massive transfusion a patient could easily receive 10–20 ml/kg within minutes.

Table 8i.3. Revised/restrictive fluid doses and rates for trauma/bleeding patients.

Fluid	Dose (ml/kg)		Time-frame	Use
Isotonic crystalloid	Dog	10–15	20–30 min	Initial "slowless"
	Cat	5–10		Repeat 1–2 times
HTS (7–7.5%) or	Dog	3–6	5–10 min	Impending CV collapse
"turbostarch"	Cat	2–4		Traumatic brain injury
Synthetic colloid	Dog	3–5	20–30 min	Blood products not available
	Cat	2–3		
Fresh whole blood	Dog	10–20	15 min to 4 h	Unresponsive to crystalloid
	Cat	7–10		Moderate/severe hemorrhage
Packed RBCs or plasma	Dog	5–10		Anemia/hypoproteinemia
	Cat	3–5		Massive transfusion

CV, cardiovascular; HTS, hypertonic saline; RBCs, red blood cells. "Turbostarch" is the 1:2 combination of 23.4% HTS and synthetic colloid.

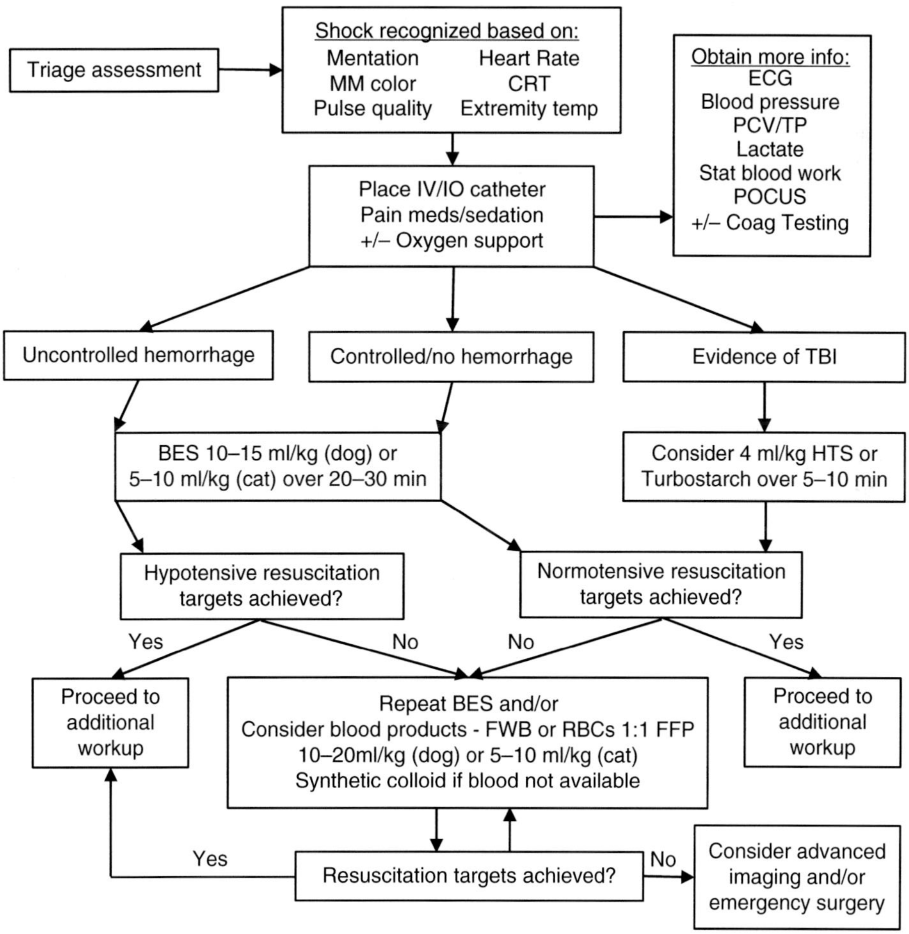

Figure 8i.2. Algorithm with suggested approach to fluid resuscitation with trauma/hemorrhage. BES, balanced electrolyte solution; CRT, capillary refill time; FFP, fresh frozen plasma; FWB, fresh whole blood; HTS, hypertonic saline; IO, intraosseous; IV, intravenous; MM, mucous membranes; PCV/TP, packed cell volume/total protein; POCUS, point-of-care ultrasound; RBCs, red blood cells. Note: "Turbostarch" is the 1:2 combination of 23.4% HTS and synthetic colloid.

8i.4 Monitoring and Resuscitation Endpoints

Many of the concepts regarding monitoring and resuscitation endpoints are similar to those discussed regarding the general approach to resuscitation (Chapter 6i). However, an important distinction exists for the patient with active/uncontrolled bleeding. As previously mentioned, aggressive resuscitative efforts could exacerbate hemorrhage, as could attempts to normalize vitals and blood pressure. It stands to reason that a sudden increase in perfusion pressure could serve to disrupt clots and encourage more bleeding to occur. This concern has brought forth the notion of **hypotensive resuscitation**, or permissive hypotension. In this approach the goal is to achieve minimally acceptable perfusion pressure, particularly with regard to vital organs (heart, brain, lung, and kidneys), until hemostasis is achieved. While there is significant debate in human medicine, and very limited evidence in veterinary medicine, it is reasonable to target a systolic blood pressure of 80–100 mm Hg, and/or a mean arterial blood pressure (MAP) of 50–70 mm Hg (Palmer and Martin, 2014). During this period, mild to moderate abnormalities in other perfusion parameters (tachycardia, pallor, prolonged capillary refill, etc.) are allowed to persist. Once hemostasis is achieved, then more normal resuscitation targets (as described in Chapter 6i) should be pursued. Ideally permissive hypotension should only be applied for a limited time (< 3–4 h), as potentially irreversible tissue ischemia could develop (Palmer and Martin, 2014). If hemostasis has not been achieved, then emergent surgical intervention is warranted.

A notable exception to the application of permissive hypotension is for patients with concurrent traumatic brain injury (TBI). Patients with increased intracranial pressure are even more dependent on MAP to maintain cerebral perfusion. As a result, allowing for lower blood pressure could serve to

Clinical Case 8i.1

A 2-year-old castrated male Labrador retriever (weighing 40 kg) presents 45 min after being hit by a car. His initial vitals are as follows:

Weight 40 kg
HR 180, RR panting, Temp 100.2
Pulse quality decreased, MM pale, CRT 3–4 sec
Normal hydration
Mentation dull
Oscillometric blood pressure – 70/40 mm Hg (mean 48 mm Hg)
Abdomen mildly distended

Based on this information you are concerned that he is in shock, most likely secondary to internal hemorrhage. While an intravenous catheter is being placed and blood is obtained, you devise an initial fluid therapy plan. Owing to immediate availability, you choose a balanced electrolyte solution (lactated Ringer's solution) to start your resuscitation. With the concern for active hemorrhage, you also elect for the revised approach regarding volume and rate:

Revised isotonic crystalloid = 10 ml/kg × 40 kg = 400 ml given over 20 min.

He is also given some pain medication (hydromorphone 0.05 mg/kg). As the slowless finishes, you reassess his vitals and have some blood work results:

HR 160, RR panting, Temp 100.7
Pulse quality moderate, MM pale pink, CRT 3 sec
Mentation QAR
Oscillometric blood pressure – 95/60 mm Hg (mean 72 mm Hg)
PCV/TP 34%, TP 5.2 g/dl (normal 37–53%, 5.6–7.1 g/dl)
Lactate 4.1 mg/dl (normal < 2 mg/dl)

Point-of-care ultrasound reveals a moderate amount of echogenic fluid, and abdominocentesis yields a hemorrhagic effusion. Based on this the suspicion of traumatic, uncontrolled hemorrhage is confirmed. His mentation has improved, and there are no signs of head trauma. In this case, application of hypotensive resuscitation is reasonable. Given that his blood pressure has reached the target range (80–100 mm Hg), it is decided not to administer an additional slowless. Instead he is placed on a maintenance rate of isotonic crystalloid and it is decided to administer aminocaproic acid (50 mg/kg loading dose followed by 15 mg/kg/h CRI for 8 h).

Re-check blood pressure 1 h later is still 100/63 (75) mm Hg, but his PCV/TP is now 27% and 4.6 g/dl. His mentation is quieter, his heart rate has increased to 170, and lactate is 4.5 mg/dl. You decide to mobilize blood products for him with a plan to give 10 ml/kg (400 ml) of fresh whole blood from your in-house donor over the next 3–4 h. Overnight he remains stable with no further need for products.

Clinical Case 8i.2

A 5-year-old FS Pug (weighing 8 kg) presents after falling from a third-story window. She was brought immediately to your veterinary clinic, which is approximately 30 min away. Here are her initial vitals:

HR 160, RR 24, Temp 97.0
PQ decreased, MM pale pink, CRT 3 sec
Laterally recumbent
Mentation dull to stuporous, anisicoria noted
Marked swelling/bruising over left proximal hind limb with crepitus and instability
Doppler blood pressure – 80 mm Hg

Based on these findings, you are concerned that she has sustained traumatic brain injury, as well as a femoral fracture with associated hemorrhage. While an intravenous catheter is being placed and blood is obtained, you devise an initial fluid therapy plan. Given the concern for increased intracranial pressure and need for volume expansion, you decide to use a low-volume resuscitation strategy:

Turbostarch dose = 3–6 ml/kg. Decide to give 4 ml/kg × 8 kg = 32 ml given over 5 min

To create turbostarch, dilute 11 ml of the 23.4% HTS stock solution with 21 ml VetStarch (1:2 dilution).

After the bolus of turbostarch her mentation improves, as do her vitals. You also obtain some additional information:

HR 150, RR 30, Temp 99.0
PQ moderate, MM pale pink, CRT 3–4 sec
Mentation dull, anisocoria resolved
Doppler blood pressure – 90 mm Hg
PCV/TP – 38%/6.0 g/dl

The patient has shown improvement but is still hypotensive. While there is concern for ongoing hemorrhage into the fracture site, the presence of TBI negates the application of hypotensive resuscitation. Instead you decide to give a cautious isotonic crystalloid slowless:

Revised isotonic crystalloid = 10 ml/kg × 8 kg = 80 ml given over 30 min.

After this administration the patient is more alert and able to sit upright. Recheck Doppler blood pressure is 110 mm Hg mm, color and CRT have also improved. Her heart rate is still 150 so you give her some pain medication (methadone 0.2 mg/kg). She is placed on a maintenance fluid rate and monitored closely overnight.

exacerbate neurological injury and worsen recovery (Palmer, 2017). In these circumstances the approach should be to achieve a more normal blood pressure, though large-volume crystalloid should still be avoided (as it could serve to worsen cerebral edema). Instead, use of HTS is recommended, with the dual purpose of increasing circulating volume/blood pressure and decreasing intracranial pressure. Early use of blood products to help optimize oxygen delivery is also recommended.

8i.5 Conclusion

Fluid resuscitation often plays a major role in the management of patients experiencing trauma and/or hemorrhage. Early recognition and categorization of bleeding can help guide decisions related to the ideal type and rate of fluid administration. Isotonic crystalloids are a reasonable starting point for most circumstances, given that they are readily available, low-cost, and reasonably effective. A revised, less-is-more approach is recommended, with the notion that a gentler approach may be more effective and less likely to exacerbate uncontrolled hemorrhage. Once resuscitation has been initiated, frequent monitoring and reassessment are needed to gauge response and determine if additional volume and/or other fluid types may be needed. Early application of blood products (if available) is recommended in patients with moderate to severe hemorrhage. In addition, the bleeding patient may warrant consideration of a hypotensive resuscitation strategy by targeting a lower blood pressure until hemostasis can be achieved. If target endpoints cannot be reached, surgical intervention may be needed. This suggested approach to fluid administration in trauma/hemorrhage is presented in Fig. 8i.2.

References

Adamik, K.-N. and Yozova, E.D. (2021) Colloids yes or no? – a "Gretchen question" answered. *Frontiers in Veterinary Science* 8, 624049.

Cooper, E.S. (2019) Pathophysiology of shock. In: Drobatz, K.J., Hopper, K., Rozanski, E. and Silverstein, D.C. (eds) *Textbook of Small Animal Emergency Medicine*. John Wiley and Sons, Hoboken, New Jersey, pp. 981–985.

Cotton, B.A., Guy, J.S., Morris, J.A. *et al.* (2006) The cellular, metabolic, and systemic consequences of aggressive fluid resuscitation strategies. *Shock* 26(2), 115–121.

Dutton, R.P. (2007) Current concepts in hemorrhagic shock. *Anesthesiology Clinics* 25, 23–34.

Hall, K. and Drobatz, K. (2021) Volume resuscitation in the acute hemorrhaging patient: historic use to current applications. *Frontiers in Veterinary Science* 8, 638104.

Lenz, A., Franklin, G.A. and Cheadle, W.G. (2007) Systemic inflammation after trauma. *Injury* 38(12), 1336–1345.

Muir, W.W. (2006) Trauma: physiology, pathophysiology, and clinical implications. *Journal of Veterinary Emergency and Critical Care* 16(4), 253–263.

Palmer, L. (2017) Fluid management in patients with trauma – restrictive vs liberal approach. *Veterinary Clinics of North America Small Animal Practice* 47, 397–410.

Palmer, L. and Martin, L. (2014) Traumatic coagulopathy – Part 1: pathophysiology and diagnosis. *Journal of Veterinary Emergency and Critical Care* 24, 63–74.

Patil, V. and Shetmahajan, M. (2014) Massive transfusion and massive transfusion protocol. *Indian Journal of Anaesthesia* 58, 590–595.

Rady, M.Y. (1994) Possible mechanisms for the interaction of peripheral somatic nerve stimulation, tissue injury, and hemorrhage in the pathophysiology of traumatic shock. *Anesthesia and Analgesia* 78, 761–765.

Santry, H.P. and Alam, H.B. (2010) Fluid resuscitation: past, present, and the future. *Shock* 33(3), 229–241.

Semler, M.W. and Kellum, J.A. (2019) Balanced crystalloid solutions. *American Journal of Respiratory and Critical Care Medicine* 199(8), 952–960.

Shakur, H., Roberts, I., Bautista, R. *et al.* (2010) Effects of tranexamic acid on death, vascular occlusive events, and blood transfusion in trauma patients with significant haemorrhage (CRASH-2): a randomised, placebo-controlled trial. *Lancet* 376, 23–32.

Stein, D.M. and Scalea, T.M. (2012) Capillary leak syndrome in trauma: what is it and what are the consequences? *Advances in Surgery* 46, 237–253.

8ii Special Considerations for Septic Patients

JULIEN GUILLAUMIN

Colorado State University, Fort Collins, Colorado, USA

Sepsis is defined as life-threatening organ dysfunction caused by a dysregulated host response to infection, according to the most recently updated definition in people (Evans *et al.*, 2021), although that definition differs significantly compared with the current veterinary definition. In both people and veterinary medicine, **septic shock** is further defined as a subset of sepsis in which particularly profound circulatory, cellular, and metabolic abnormalities are associated with a greater risk of mortality than with sepsis alone (Evans *et al.*, 2021). Septic shock is caused by a combination of hypovolemia, vasodilation and cellular-metabolic disturbances, and will often require vasopressors after intravascular volume replacement. This is clinically recognized as a **septic patient** whose blood pressure is not responsive to fluid therapy alone. Owing to the complex pathophysiology, septic patients can be relatively challenging to manage with regard to fluid therapy. As seen in the case below, fluid losses in septic patients can come from various compartments and should be replaced by various types of fluid.

Hypovolemia is common in septic patients and can occur secondary to fluid loss through gastrointestinal system or third spacing, a lack of intake, and extravasation of intravascular fluid secondary to increased vascular permeability. As such, shock associated with sepsis should be treated first to restore intravascular fluid volume. **Isotonic fluid** is a logical first line of defense dealing with critically ill pets, and indeed a conservative amount of isotonic crystalloid (up to 30 ml/kg intravenous within the first hour of diagnosis) is recommended in septic shock patients (see Chapter 6i regarding fluid resuscitation). A balanced electrolyte solution such as lactate-based or acetate/gluconate-based fluid is recommended.

However, selected circumstances may require the clinician to switch to a **colloidal solution**, especially if the patient being resuscitated has developed hypoproteinemia/hypoalbuminemia or shows signs of interstitial edema. In these circumstances of decreased oncotic pressure (see Chapters 2 and 4ii), a large volume of isotonic crystalloids may be less effective at expanding the vascular volume and actually serve to worsen hypoalbuminemia and interstitial edema.

In sepsis, **albumin** is being "consumed" during the inflammatory process so the decrease in albumin levels seen after resuscitation with isotonic crystalloid can be more pronounced than expected. Incorporating plasma products as a source of species-specific albumin has been recommended in septic people, especially in septic shock cases (Finfer *et al.*, 2011; Caironi *et al.*, 2014). That recommendation can be translated to dogs and cats. Species-specific albumin can be sourced using lyophilized albumin, fresh frozen plasma (FFP) or cryo-poor plasma (CPP), depending on availability. The dose of albumin in septic patients is unknown. In people, a fixed dose is used, between 0.6–0.8 g/kg/day, and may depend on the patient's albumin level (i.e., albumin-targeted). Different formulas have been published in veterinary medicine, but they contradict each other, and their origins are unclear (see Chapter 6ii). Therefore, the author recommends a fixed dose of albumin for septic patients.

The volume of albumin given depends on the dose and concentration of the albumin product used. Lyophilized canine albumin can be diluted to a 16% solution, which contains albumin at 160 mg/ml. Plasma products such as FFP and CPP contain 29 mg/ml and 32 mg/ml of plasma product, respectively (Culler *et al.*, 2017).

DOI: 10.1079/9781789243406.0082

As the recommended dose in the septic patient is around 0.7 g/kg/day, it is easy to calculate the volume needed depending on the blood product used, and divide it by 24 h, administered as a continuous rate infusion (CRI). In a retrospective study of ten hypoalbuminemic dogs, it was shown that CPP at 1.8 ml/kg/h, corresponding to canine albumin at 1.4 g/kg/day, was associated with a rise of albumin from 1.5 g/dl to 2.1 g/dl (Culler *et al.*, 2019). The use of synthetic colloids, such as hydroxyethyl starches or gelatin, is controversial, and has generally fallen out of favor for patients with sepsis (Montealegre and Lyons, 2021). Similarly, the use of human serum albumin, although providing cost-effective, highly concentrated albumin, is controversial due to the risks of severe transfusion reactions (Montealegre and Lyons, 2021). It has been shown that canine-specific albumin increases albumin levels and colloid osmotic pressure in dogs with septic peritonitis with minimal side effects (Craft and Powell, 2012).

Clinicians should treat dehydration carefully in septic dogs and cats. The combination of hypoalbuminemia and increased vascular permeability in sepsis can lead to increased fluid extravasation when using an isotonic crystalloid. Therefore, the dehydration should be corrected more slowly compared with a normal dog or cat. Monitoring for signs of worsening interstitial edema should be more frequent, and clinicians may want to incorporate natural colloidal solutions in order to help with oncotic pressure and retention of fluid within the intravascular compartment.

The same concept can be applied to ongoing losses, depending on the source of sepsis. For example, septic peritonitis treated post-operatively with active drainage collection systems can have significant abdominal effusion and losses. The abdominal fluid protein content can be measured or estimated based on refractometry. This volume can be corrected with a combination of isotonic crystalloids and natural colloids.

In sepsis and septic shock, there are many facets of patient stabilization and treatment that need to occur in addition to the role of fluid therapy. Extensive review of sepsis management is beyond the scope of this section. Briefly, sepsis management guidelines in people (Evans *et al.*, 2021), and typically applied to dogs and cats, recommend early antibiotic therapy and early source identification and control (such as surgery in case of septic peritonitis or pyometra). As mentioned previously, septic dogs and cats who stay **hypotensive** (defined as a mean blood pressure below 65 mm Hg) despite "appropriate" intravascular fluid replacement are considered to be in septic shock. In those specific clinical scenarios, early vasopressor therapy, specifically norepinephrine, should be instituted. If norepinephrine is not available, then epinephrine as a constant rate infusion is recommended in people (Evans *et al.*, 2021).

Clinical Case 8ii.1

You are presented with a 5-year-old, 5 kg intact female mixed-breed dog who is not doing well.

History: She has a history of acute onset of vomiting, bloody diarrhea, and lethargy for the past 24 h. She has no history of coughing or sneezing, no travel history, no tick exposure. She was eating and drinking normally prior to acute illness. She is a rescue dog that lives in a foster home, stays inside, goes out to a fenced yard, and is currently on vaccines. She has been on a tapering dose of steroids for a chronic skin infection.

Physical examination: Her physical examination revealed a lateral recumbency with marked obtundation, a temperature of 103.7°F (39.8°C), a pulse rate of 160 bpm, a respiratory rate of 50/min. She appears 8% dehydrated, with weak femoral pulses, pale mucous membranes, and a capillary refill time of 4 seconds. She has no heart murmur, normal bronchovesicular sound in all quadrants, and is eupneic. Her abdomen is distended and painful, with mucopurulent vulvar discharge.

Initial assessment: Your initial assessment is some physical examination signs of shock and moderate to marked dehydration, with some gastrointestinal signs. You instruct your veterinary staff to place an intravenous catheter and get a minimal database that consists of a packed cell volume/total protein, venous blood gas and electrolytes, complete blood count, biochemistry, and blood pressure obtained by the Doppler method.

Continued

Clinical Case 8ii.1 Continued.

The diagnostic tests and their pertinent results are as follows:

Venous blood gas and electrolytes	
Packed cell volume	35%*
Total protein	6.5 g/dl
Na^+	135.8 mmol/l*
K^+	4.1 mmol/l
Cl^-	115.7 mmol/l
Lactate	6.3 mmol/l*
Hb	11.8 g/dl
Complete blood count	
Platelet count	215 × 10^9/l
Total leukocytes	5.9 × 10^9/l
Bands neutrophils	0.7 × 10^9/l (11%) *
Seg neutrophils	4.1 × 10^9/l (70%)
Lymphocytes	0.5 × 10^9/l (8%) *
Monocytes	0.4 × 10^9/l (7%)
Eosinophils	0.2 × 10^9/l (4%)
Biochemistry profile	
BUN	45 mg/dl
Creatinine	2.0 mg/dl
Phosphorus	13.2 mg/dl
Cholesterol	532 mg/dl *
Bilirubin	0.17 mg/dl
Total protein	5.3 g/dl
Albumin	2.8 g/dl *
Globulin	2.5 g/dl
Glucose	82 mg/dl
Blood pressure	
Doppler BP	40 mm Hg

*Abnormal value, outside the reference range.

Your minimal database confirmed your initial assessment of shock and dehydration. The dog is in hypotensive, hypovolemic shock and dehydrated. She has a mild hyponatremia, probably secondary to ADH secretion triggered by hypovolemia (see Chapter 8vi). She is also anemic, and while the total protein is in the normal range, with 8% dehydration it can be expected that this will decrease with rehydration.

While you continue to investigate the case, you make the decision to start intravenous fluids and answer the following three questions:

Which fluid?	An isotonic crystalloid makes the most sense here. You have a hypovolemic and dehydrated dog, and so this fluid type will help to correct both
How much?	Given the severity of this patient's shock (late decompensated), the "classic" approach to resuscitation would be reasonable. The total "shock dose" of crystalloid for a 5 kg dog is 350–500 ml (70–90 ml/kg). Resuscitation is started with one-quarter of the total shock dose (20 ml/kg), or 100 ml
How fast?	A volume of 100 ml of isotonic crystalloid can easily be given over 15–20 min

A few comments

1. Although the dog has a mild hyponatremia, there is no need to reach for a high-sodium-content fluid. On the contrary, giving a bolus of high-sodium-content fluid to a hyponatremic dog can lead to a faster-than-recommended correction of hyponatremia (see Chapter 8vi). If boluses of fluids are given to a dysnatremic patient, it is best to match the sodium concentration of the fluid to sodium concentration of the dog, within 10 mmol/l. In this specific case, a fluid containing sodium between 125 and 145 mmol/l is best.
2. Do not worry about the impact of fluid expansion on the hematocrit. Although the hematocrit may drop following resuscitation, it would only drop to the level revealed by appropriate volume expansion. Although blood is important, blood volume is more important in the acute stages.
3. The extracellular volume deficit of a 5 kg dog who is 8% dehydrated is also 400 ml, the same as a "shock" dose. However, it is important to recognize that the speed of rehydration should be much slower compared with intravascular fluid volume resuscitation.
4. Because of the low blood pressure and the high lactate, it is probable that one single one-quarter shock dose of crystalloid would not be enough. Additional boluses may be needed.

Follow up: The first crystalloid bolus mildly improves the heart rate and mentation. You elect to provide another one-quarter shock dose (100 ml) over 20 min. During this time, you perform an abdominal

Continued

Clinical Case 8ii.1 Continued.

point-of-care ultrasound and diagnose this dog with a pyometra and suspected sepsis. Her heart rate and mentation does improve with the second bolus, and her blood pressure improves to 90–100 mm Hg with Doppler. Blood work is rechecked with the PCV at 28% and total protein down to 4.3 g/dl.

At this point, the patient is anemic, hypoproteinemic, dehydrated, and in septic shock with a need for surgical intervention. In addition to source control with surgery to remove the source of sepsis, broad-spectrum antibiotics (ampicillin/sulbactam and enrofloxacin) are given intravenously.

While waiting to go to surgery, the patient declines again. Heart rate has increased, mentation has declined, and Doppler blood pressure is down to 50–60 mm Hg. With regard to further resuscitation, the patient has already received isotonic crystalloid at 40 ml/kg (half of total shock dose), and so additional administration is unlikely to be beneficial. Especially given the patient's hypoalbuminemia, it is decided to give a bolus of natural colloid (FFP at 4 ml/kg over 20–30 min) while also starting norepinephrine as a vasopressor.

The combination of these interventions helps to stabilize the patient and she is taken to surgery. Upon returning, her blood pressure and vitals have remained adequate. At this point fluid therapy is geared toward replacement of her dehydration and providing oncotic support. As the dog is already receiving 200 ml out of the 400 ml deficit (8% dehydration × 5 kg = 400 ml), the remaining 200 ml is given over 12 h (17 ml/h) along with maintenance fluid rate (using the allometric formula of $132 \times BW^{0.75}$ (kg), the maintenance rate is 18 ml/h). So she is placed on isotonic crystalloid at 35 ml/h.

It is also decided to start her on a CRI of FFP at 1–2 ml/kg/h to help replace albumin and provide oncotic support. Over the next 48 h she is successfully weaned from pressors and the plasma CRI, and transitioned to a maintenance fluid rate by the time of discharge.

References

Caironi, P., Tognoni, G., Masson, S. *et al.* (2014) Albumin replacement in patients with severe sepsis or septic shock. *New England Journal of Medicine* 370, 1412–1421.

Craft, E.M. and Powell, L.L. (2012) The use of canine-specific albumin in dogs with septic peritonitis. *Journal of Veterinary Emergency and Critical Care* 22(6), 631–639.

Culler, C.A., Iazbik, C. and Guillaumin, J. (2017) Comparison of albumin, colloid osmotic pressure, von Willebrand factor, and coagulation factors in canine cryopoor plasma, cryoprecipitate, and fresh frozen plasma. *Journal of Veterinary Emergency and Critical Care* 27(6), 638–644.

Culler, C.A., Balakrishnan, A., Yaxley, P.E. *et al.* (2019) Clinical use of cryopoor plasma continuous rate infusion in critically ill, hypoalbuminemic dogs. *Journal of Veterinary Emergency and Critical Care* 29(3), 314–320.

Evans, L., Rhodes, A., Alhazzani, W. *et al.* (2021) Surviving sepsis campaign: international guidelines for management of sepsis and septic shock. *Intensive Care Medicine* 47(11), 1181–1247.

Finfer, S., McEvoy, S., Bellomo, R. *et al.* (2011) Impact of albumin compared to saline on organ function and mortality of patients with severe sepsis. *Intensive Care Medicine* 37, 86–96.

Montealegre, F. and Lyons, B.M. (2021) Fluid therapy in dogs and cats with sepsis. *Frontiers in Veterinary Science* 258, 622127.

8iii Impact of Heart Disease on Fluid Therapy

JIWOONG HER

The Ohio State University, Columbus, Ohio, USA

Patients with heart disease are not ideal candidates for fluid administration. However, some patients with heart disease develop situations that may necessitate fluid therapy (e.g., dehydration). Another indication is to help deliver continuous infusions of intravenous medications that would otherwise have a very low rate of administration (such as vasopressors, inotrope, anti-arrhythmic agents, or analgesia). In patients with heart disease, correcting fluid deficit and preventing fluid overload can sometimes be challenging. Before planning fluid therapy, it is recommended to obtain baseline information, including body weight, packed cell volume, total solid, urine specific gravity, and kidney values. Imaging modalities such as radiography and echocardiography are warranted to fully diagnose and stage the patient's heart disease. This may be particularly important in patients that have a heart murmur but the extent of structural heart disease is not known. Following fluid administration, serial evaluation of the patient is required to determine the response to fluid therapy and to monitor clinical signs for volume overload.

As heart disease progresses, several counter-regulatory mechanisms are activated to maintain circulating volume at the expense of increase in total body water (Cooke and Snyder, 1998). Overall, these neuroendocrine mechanisms promote sodium and water retention. Therefore, fluid selection for these patients should be made with awareness of sodium content. With this in mind, the fluid of choice for patients with heart disease is ideally a hypotonic fluid (see Chapter 3). Utilizing either 0.45% NaCl + 2.5% dextrose or 5% dextrose, supplemented with potassium chloride as needed (see Chapter 7ii), is recommended when fluid therapy is indicated for patients with advanced cardiac disease and no current signs of heart failure (Bonagura *et al.*, 2012). Caution should be exercised when using hypotonic fluids, as these may lead to water retention and subsequent hyponatremia (Hansen and Vigani, 2017). Serial monitoring of serum electrolytes is recommended to then allow treatment adjustments. If the patient has minimal radiographic or echocardiographic changes, isotonic fluids (e.g., lactated Ringer's solution, Normosol-R, Plasma-Lyte 148) may be indicated to carefully replace volume (presuming isotonic losses). Among isotonic crystalloids, lactated Ringer's solution may be preferred because it has the lowest osmolarity and lowest sodium concentration (130 mEq/l) compared with other isotonic crystalloids. Short-term administration of isotonic crystalloids may be well tolerated in patients with mild cardiac disease, provided the volume and rate of fluid therapy are chosen carefully.

The rate of fluid therapy administration is just as important as the type of fluid administered. The degree of physical, radiographic, and echocardiographic changes guides the initial rate of fluid therapy. A general rule is to decrease the fluid rate to approximately one-third to one-half of the rate for a healthy patient. For example, when calculating replacement fluid rates, it would be recommended to replace dehydration over a longer period of time (for example, 24–36 h rather than 12–18 h).

The best way to approach fluid therapy in patients with heart disease is to avoid fluid overload in the first place. To aid in this regard, exercise caution when using an isotonic crystalloid fluid bolus for hypotensive patients with heart disease, as they may not be able to tolerate rapidly increased hydrostatic pressure created by a high rate of fluid. For hypotensive patients with significant heart disease, avoid using hypertonic solutions (e.g., 3–7.5% hypertonic saline) or colloids (e.g., VetStarch), because this can lead to rapid intravascular volume

DOI: 10.1079/9781789243406.0083

expansion and subsequent development of interstitial edema (e.g., pulmonary edema) or third spacing (e.g., pleural effusion, ascites). Instead, using a positive inotrope (e.g., dobutamine) to increase contractility may be the preferred choice over fluids, to avoid fluid overload and to maintain cardiac output and tissue perfusion.

Patients with heart disease require careful, serial evaluation of hydration and perfusion parameters, body weight, and hemodynamic variables. Signs of fluid overload can include tachypnea, increased respiratory rate and effort, cough, tachycardia, newly developed heart murmur, pulmonary crackles, ascites, serous nasal discharge, and chemosis (Fig. 8iii.1). If fluid overload is suspected, the first step is to discontinue intravenous fluid administration. Oxygen supplementation and furosemide can be given until clinical improvement is noted. Radiography and echocardiography can provide evidence of pulmonary edema and volume overload (Fig. 8iii.2). From there further adjustment and a more cautious approach to fluid administration may then proceed.

If the risk of fluid overload due to direct intravascular volume expansion is too high, another option is to use free-choice water-by-mouth or administration of water via nasogastric/nasoesophageal tube. These tubes are easily placed in patients with heart disease, because they do not require general anesthesia or heavy sedation. Enteral fluid therapy avoids the risk of fluid overload associated with intravenous fluid administration, because the gastrointestinal tract can remove excess water. Therefore, if used in conjunction with intravenous fluid or alone, enteral fluid therapy is useful for the treatment of dehydration and electrolyte loss in

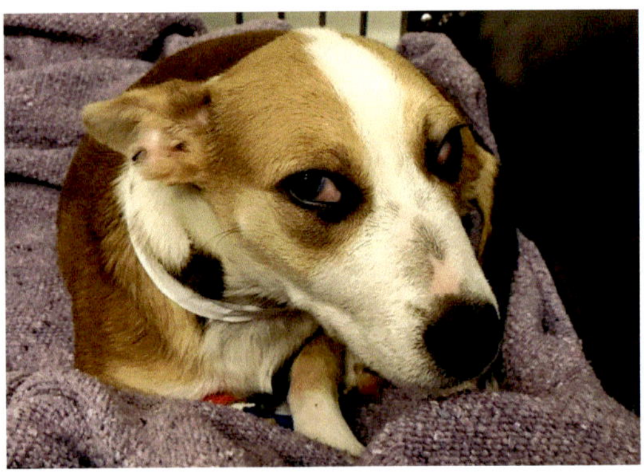

Fig. 8iii.1. Conjunctival edema (chemosis) due to fluid overload from excessive fluid administration.

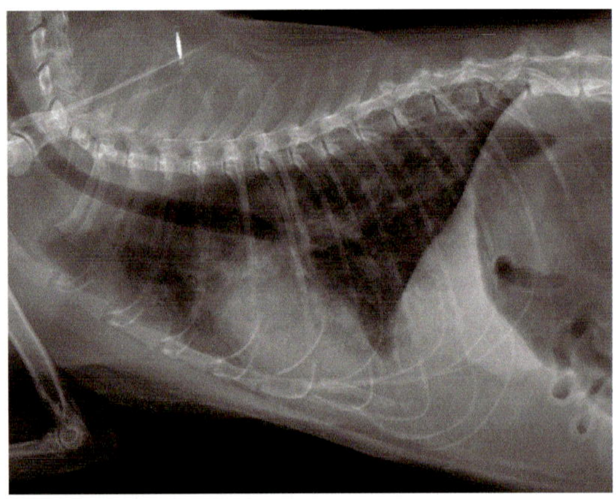

Fig. 8iii.2. Right lateral thoracic radiograph of a feline patient with left-sided congestive heart failure.

Clinical Case 8iii.1

A 4-year-old, 10 kg male neutered Cavalier King Charles Spaniel is presented to your clinic for vomiting, diarrhea, and anorexia for 24 h. On presentation, the patient is quiet, alert, and responsive. He is estimated to be 5% dehydrated on presentation. Physical examination reveals grade 2/6 systolic apical heart murmur with fair, synchronous femoral pulses. Chest radiographs show mild left atrial enlargement but no changes in pulmonary vasculature. In determining his fluid therapy plan, you want to replace his deficit, but minimize the risk of causing fluid overload. Here is an example of how those calculations could be performed:

Fluid deficit = (10 kg × 0.05 × 1000 ml = 500 ml) over 36 h = 14 ml/h
Maintenance rate = 132 × (10)0.75/24 h = 31 ml/h
Total = 45 ml [maintenance-type fluid (e.g. 0.45% NaCl) at 31 ml/h + replacement-type fluid (e.g., LRS) at 14 ml/h] over the next 36 h.

Note: It was decided to use hypotonic solution for maintenance rate and isotonic solution for fluid deficit, and to replace fluid deficit slowly over 36 h instead of 24 h, due to concerns of mitral valve disease.

Clinical Case 8iii.2

A 10-year-old, 8 kg neutered male Miniature Schnauzer is presented to your clinic for diarrhea and anorexia for 24 h. The patient is estimated to have 5% dehydration on physical examination. On presentation, the patient is quiet, alert, and responsive. Physical examination reveals grade 5/6 systolic apical heart murmur with fair, synchronous femoral pulses. The patient was seen by a cardiologist a few months ago for congestive heart failure. Since then, he has been treated with pimobendan, furosemide, and enalapril for mitral valve disease. With these factors in mind, here is a potential approach to providing fluid therapy:

Fluid deficit = (8 kg × 0.05 × 1,000 ml = 400 ml) over 36 h = 11 ml/h

Maintenance volume = $132 \times (8)^{0.75}/24$ h = 26 ml/h

While the patient is still receiving cardiac medications, water at 26 ml/h (maintenance rate) is administered via nasogastric tube for the first 8–12 h. Even though the fluid deficit is estimated to be 400 ml, it is decided to hold on to replace the volume and to start him with appetite stimulant instead. The plan is to increase the nasogastric fluid rate from 26 (maintenance) to 37 ml/h (maintenance rate + fluid deficit) if the patient tolerates the starting rate but remains anorexic.

patients with heart disease. If the patient receives enteral nutrition, water content in the nutrition should be included in the total water intakes to avoid over supplementation of daily fluid.

References

Bonagura, J.D., Lehmkuhl, L.B. and Autran de Morais, H. (2012) Fluid and diuretic therapy in heart failure. In: DiBartola, S.P. (ed.) *Fluid, Electrolyte, and Acid-Base Disorders in Small Animal Practice*, 4th edn. W.B. Saunders, St Louis, Missouri, pp. 514–543.

Cooke, K.L. and Snyder, P.S. (1998) Fluid therapy in the cardiac patient. *Veterinary Clinics of North America. Small Animal Practice* 28(3), 663–676.

Hansen, B. and Vigani, A. (2017) Maintenance fluid therapy: isotonic versus hypotonic solutions. *Veterinary Clinics of North America. Small Animal Practice* 47(2), 383–395.

8iv Impact of Renal Disease on Fluid Therapy

ANDA YOUNG

The Ohio State University, Columbus, Ohio, USA

Acute kidney injury (AKI) is characterized by a continuum of functional and/or parenchymal damage resulting in systemic accumulation of metabolic toxins. It is defined as clinically documentable when there is an acute increase in creatinine by 0.3 mg/dl within 48 h or oliguric urine output characterized as <0.5–1 ml/kg/h over 6 h (Khwaja, 2012; Cowgill, 2016). Normal urine output (i.e., 1–2 ml/kg/h) or **polyuria**, characterized as >2 ml/kg/h, may also be seen at any stage of acute kidney injury, depending on the etiology and location of kidney injury (Khwaja, 2012). Acute kidney injury and fluids are closely linked, as hypovolemia is a major risk factor for the development of AKI (Perner *et al.*, 2017). The rationale for fluid therapy in the prevention or treatment of acute kidney injury is to optimize intravascular circulating volume, cardiac output, renal blood flow (RBF), and glomerular filtrate rate (GFR), the primary determinant of uremic toxin excretion (Perner *et al.*, 2017; Ostermann *et al.*, 2019). In the face of AKI, it is an oversimplification to say that increased RBF leads to increased GFR. The discordance between RBF and GFR has led the critical care community to avoid "one size fits all" fluid management and reassess the role fluid therapy plays in the management of acute kidney injury. The conundrum faced by a number of clinicians is about what significance dehydration is playing in the pathogenesis and degree of azotemia (how much is pre-renal versus renal). Said another way, does the elevation in creatinine and reduced urine output reflect severe dehydration and hypovolemia or has renal injury occurred leading to reduced renal functionality and a state of intrinsic oliguria or anuria? This becomes important, as intrinsic renal failure may make a patient intolerant to even moderate amounts of fluid therapy. This question has historically been addressed through assessment of urine specific gravity and/or urine sodium concentration which, when normal, would suggest intact tubular function. This approach may be reliable in most circumstances, but such urine parameters may be less reliable in cases of early renal injury, glomerulonephritis or sepsis-induced AKI (Khwaja, 2012).

The aforementioned scenarios introduce the most emphasized point, which is patient hydration assessment and frequent reassessment. Overzealous fluid administration may only worsen renal function through mechanisms of increased workload to the kidneys, increased oxygen/energy consumption, interstitial edema, and/or alterations in renal microvasculature, which further alters renal blood flow. Because risk of harm exists, being in a state of dehydration or overhydration, frequent patient assessment of hydration status using subjective and objective parameters is strongly recommended. Additionally, measurement of urine output should be considered as a tool to monitor trends in urine production and as a means to ensure that the fluid therapy being administered is not insufficient or in excess of that which the patient produces (Fig. 8iv.1).

Because patients with acute kidney injury often enter a state of polyuria consisting of losses that are isotonic to the patient, isotonic replacement fluids are often selected (i.e., 0.9% NaCl, P-lyte, LRS). That being said, isotonic solutions often have an excess of sodium and chloride that far exceeds patient daily maintenance requirements (see Chapter 6iii). Excess chloride reaching the distal tubule of the nephron leads to tubuloglomerular feedback and imbalances between vascular tone of the afferent and efferent glomerular arterioles, with consequences of reduced GFR and reduced renal blood flow. This salt-induced renal injury is termed **sodium glomerulopathy** (Aviv *et al.*, 2004). This

DOI: 10.1079/9781789243406.0084

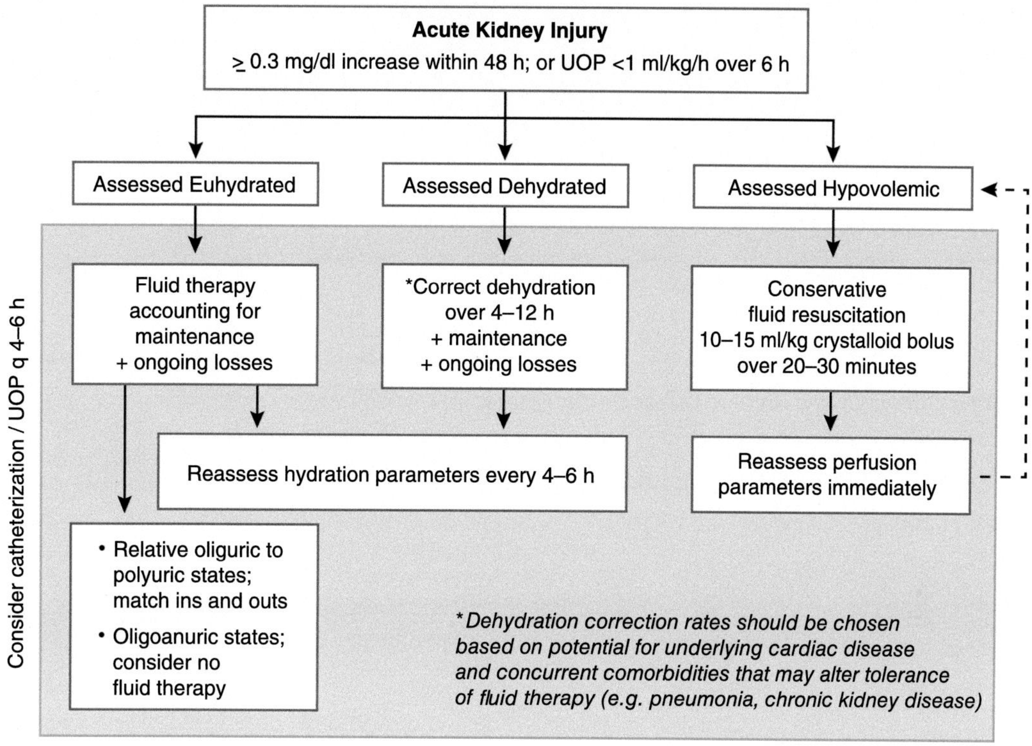

Fig. 8iv.1. A clinical approach to the management of fluid therapy in the acute kidney patient. (© The Ohio State University.)

pathophysiology is relevant, as 0.9% NaCl has been shown in human literature to increase risk of AKI, morbidity and mortality as compared with balanced solutions (Rein and Coca, 2019). Recent prospective observational studies have evaluated the risk of hospital-acquired AKI in hospitalized canine patients receiving balanced crystalloids (e.g., Plasma-Lyte A, LRS); 25% of patients developed AKI (Libin *et al.*, 2020). Statistically significant risk factors for developing AKI included elevated blood pressure at presentation and the maximum corrected chloride value, with higher chloride correlating to higher risk for AKI. In this same study, total crystalloid volume on a ml/kg basis was significantly higher in the hyperchloremic group, thus it is not discerned whether a positive fluid balance was a contributor to the development of AKI (Libin *et al.*, 2020). Limitations of the previous study limit the ability to draw conclusions regarding causal effect; however, in patients with established AKI or chronic kidney disease or who are deemed to be at risk for the development of AKI, it is warranted to avoid crystalloid fluids containing supraphysiologic levels of chloride (i.e., 0.9% NaCl) and monitor hydration/volume status and chloride levels regularly in an effort to avoid deleterious effects of crystalloid fluid therapy on the kidneys.

Isotonic crystalloids continue to be accepted as first-line therapy in patients with renal disease, but the most appropriate crystalloid for use in AKI remains to be established (Young *et al*,, 2015; Perner *et al.*, 2017; Self *et al.*, 2018). During initial phases of treatment, balanced crystalloids are recommended due to their physiologic chloride levels and tonicity that mimic patient urinary losses (Langston, 2017). With this in mind, fluid therapy in patients with renal disease can be divided into three phases: (i) resuscitation; (ii) maintenance; and (iii) reduction/removal (Goldstein, 2014). Until further evidence is presented, balanced crystalloids continue to be an acceptable choice for all phases whilst being cognizant of patient serum chloride levels.

Resuscitation measures are indicated in dehydrated and hypovolemic patients who are living on the spectrum of pre-renal azotemia transitioning to ischemic renal injury and acute tubular necrosis (Goldstein, 2014). Strategies for assessment are outlined in Fig. 8iv.1 with the goal of achieving effective circulating volume and enhancing end organ perfusion. The volume and speed at which crystalloids are administered during this phase will be based on clinical assessment. Patients assessed to be hypovolemic may require "shock" doses of balanced crystalloids (dog: 10–20 ml/kg over 20–30 min; cat: 5–10 ml/kg over 20–30 min) (see Chapter 6i). Patients assessed to be dehydrated can have their fluid deficit corrected over 8–24 h. Slower rates of correction may be chosen for patients who suffer from chronic dehydration or lack tolerance of high rates of crystalloid administration (i.e., pneumonia, known/occult heart disease). The dehydration deficit can be calculated with the following formula (see also Chapter 6ii):

Body weight (kg) × estimated % dehydration = fluid deficit (l)

Following resuscitation and replacement, the patient enters the **maintenance** phase, where fluid therapy and nutrition are provided to target a state of euhydration. The volumes and rates at which crystalloids are administered during this phase will be based on the patient's voluntary intake as it compares with the patient's involuntary losses. At this phase it is most important to observe for states of polyuria, oliguria, anuria, weight gain/loss, and fluid overload. These observations may dictate decreasing or increasing fluid rates with the goal of maintaining euhydration and avoiding a positive fluid balance and fluid overload, as this increases the workload on the kidneys and is associated with higher mortality. Monitoring of urine output with an indwelling urinary catheter and closed collection system can be extremely helpful during this phase. Once a status of euhydration is achieved, the clinician can match "ins and outs" (i.e., fluid rate = hourly urine output), which limits the margin of error as it provides an automatic adjustment for polyuric or oliguric states—states that do not follow the rules of classical "maintenance" fluid therapy formulas. The logarithmic formulas for maintenance fluid therapy provided below are more accurate for variable patient sizes (i.e., the same formula can be used for Chihuahua as for Great Dane) (see also Chapter 6iii):

Dog: Lean body weight (kg) 0.75 × 132 = daily fluid requirement (ml/day)
Cat: Lean body weight (kg) 0.75 × 70 = daily fluid requirement (ml/day)

Removal of fluid therapy is typically never emergent, the exception being the fluid-overloaded patient. Once to twice-daily monitoring of renal values is essential to assess for spikes or a plateau in creatinine values. The creatinine plateau may or may not be within reference range; however, the actual value is less important, as it may takes weeks to months before full renal recovery is observed. Once a plateau is reached, if hydration parameters are stable, a nutritional plan has been established and the patient is not suffering from excessive losses (e.g., severe polyuria, severe diarrhea), a gradual fluid taper may commence. Fluid rates can be decreased by approximately 25% every 24 h (Langston, 2017). A patient is considered to be successfully responding to a fluid taper if they are able to maintain their hydration through enteral routes and do not experience significant weight loss or jumps in their creatinine values. Fluid tapering may occur over the course of 2–3 days and the clinician may elect to measure a creatinine with the patient being on no fluid therapy for 24 h, to establish a baseline for future monitoring. Clients who experience financial stress due to the significant costs associated with AKI or acute or chronic kidney disease should be educated early about esophageal

Clinical Case 8iv.1

A 6-year-old FS mixed-breed dog weighing 12 kg presents with a 3-day history of progressive inappetence, increased thirst, urinary accidents in the home and one episode of vomiting. The patient has no pertinent medical history and had a normal chemistry panel performed 3 months ago at her annual veterinary visit. Other pertinent history is that the patient roams a wooded yard and has a history of drinking stagnant water. The patient is in good body condition and has a generally unremarkable physical examination aside from general malaise. She is assessed to be 7% dehydrated but is deemed cardiovascularly stable. The following chemistry panel is obtained at the time of presentation.

Continued

Clinical Case 8iv.1 Continued.

Parameter	Value	S.I. (US)	Reference low	Reference high
Hematocrit	57	%	40	59
Plasma protein	(7.9)	g/l (g/dl)	56 (5.6)	73 (7.3)
BUN	46.4 (130)	mmol/l (mg/dl)	3.57 (10)	9.64 (27)
Creatinine	427 (5.6)	μmol/l (mg/dl)	7.63 (0.1)	99.1 (1.3)
Phosphorus	2.39 (7.4)	mmol/l (mg/dl)	0.71 (2.2)	2.03 (6.3)
Calcium – total	2.13 (8.5)	mmol/l (mg/dl)	2.27 (9.1)	2.88 (11.5)
Sodium	141 (141)	mmol/l (mEq/l)	145 (145)	154 (154)
Potassium	3.5 (2.5)	mol/l (mEq/l)	3.9 (3.9)	5.5 (5.5)
Chloride	113 (113)	mmol/l (mEq/l)	107 (107)	118 (118)
Anion Gap	29 (29)	Mmol/l (mEq/l)	15 (15)	25 (25)
Osmolality (calc)	326 (326)	mmol/kg (mOsm/kg)	289 (289)	308 (308)
Bicarbonate – total	14.1 (14.1)	mmol/l (mEq/l)	18 (18)	27 (27)
ALT – alanine amino transferase	2 (120)	μkat/l (IU/l)	0.3 (18)	1.8 (108)
AST – aspartate amino transferase	1.14 (68)	μkat/l (IU/l)	0.27 (16)	0.85 (51)
AP – alkaline phosphatase	2.5 (150)	μkat/l (IU/l)	0.2 (12)	2.22 (133)
CK – creatine kinase	3.16 (189)	μkat/l (IU/l)	0.89 (53)	6.21 (372)
Cholesterol	5.28 (240)	mmol/l (mg/dl)	3.16 (122)	8.94 (345)
Bilirubin – total	6.84 (0.4)	μmol/l (mg/dl)	0.86 (0.5)	3.42 (0.2)
Total protein – Serum	80 (8.0)	g/l (g/dl)	51 (5.1)	71 (7.1)
Albumin	31 (3.1)	g/l (g/dl)	33 (3.3)	42 (4.2)
Globulin	24 (2.4)	g/l (g/dl)	17 (1.7)	34 (3.4)
A/G ratio	13 (1.3)	g/l (g/dl)	0 (0)	0 (0)
Glucose – Serum	7.44 (134)	mmol/l (mg/dl)	3.72 (67)	7.05 (127)
GGT	0.08 (5.00)	μkat/l (IU/l)	0 (0)	0.37 (22.3)

Urine is collected via cystocentesis for urinalysis and culture. An abdominal ultrasound is performed which is generally unremarkable (i.e., kidneys show normal architecture), but the urinary bladder is small. Given the history, leptospirosis microagglutination titers are submitted. The patient is diagnosed with an acute kidney injury and admitted to the small animal ICU for IV fluid therapy and monitoring. The patient is started on doxycycline 5 mg/kg IV q12h in the interim. The following calculations are used to generate her initial replacement fluid therapy plan using an isotonic crystalloid:

1. 7% dehydration fluid deficit:
   12 kg × 0.07 = 0.840 l deficit
   840 ml ÷ 12 h = 70 ml/h
2. Maintenance fluid rate:
   12 kg0.75 × 132 = 851 ml/day ÷ 24 h/day = 35 ml/h
3. Total fluid rate:
   70 ml/h + 35 ml/h = 105 ml/h for 12 h

Given that the patient was noted to have a small urinary bladder during ultrasound examination, a urinary catheter is placed and attached to a closed collection set. Total urine output is measured every 4 h. The patient's hydration status is assessed 4 h after starting fluid therapy, at which point she is deemed to be still mildly dehydrated. Fluid therapy is continued as previously calculated.

Hydration status is assessed again 8 h after starting fluid therapy, at which time she is deemed to be euhydrated and has gained approximately 7% of her body weight. Urine output data is analyzed.

1. Total urine output at 4 h:
   48 ml over 4 h = 12 ml/h (1 ml/kg/h)
2. Total urine output at 8 h:
   56 ml over 4 h = 14 ml/h (1.2 ml/kg/h)

Because the patient has gained weight, is euhydrated and exhibiting signs of relative oliguria, a fluid rate is chosen that matches her outs so as not to add excessive volume that will not be tolerated, resulting in a state of fluid overload. As such the patient is placed on 14 ml/h and this rate will be adjusted accordingly every 4 h to match her next urine output measurement, provided that the patient maintains a euhydrated state. Note that while technically this is below her normal maintenance rate (35 ml/h), based on her urine output that rate would be more fluids than she needs. It would also be reasonable to consider switching her to a maintenance-type fluid (e.g., 0.45% NaCl). A creatinine value will be obtained every 12 h and a body weight will be obtained every 8 h to monitor for trends and response to therapy.

feeding tubes, as these can often provide an "exit strategy" to get patients home sooner so that they can continue to receive supportive care medications (e.g., antiemetics, phosphorus binders), nutrition, and hydration. Owner education is prudent, to ensure that family members are willing and able to provide this essential nursing care that can provide significant support through the renal recovery phase.

References

Aviv, A., Hollenberg, N.K. and Weder, A.B. (2004) Sodium glomerulopathy: tubuloglomerular feedback and renal injury in African Americans. *Kidney International* 65, 361–368.

Cowgill, L. (2016) Grading of acute kidney injury. International Renal Interest Society (IRIS). Available at: http://www.iris-kidney.com/guidelines/grading.html (accessed August 2022).

Goldstein, S.L. (2014) Fluid management in acute kidney injury. *Journal of Intensive Care Medicine* 29, 183–189.

Khwaja, A. (2012) KDIGO clinical practice guidelines for acute kidney injury. *Nephron Clinical Practice* 120, c179–184.

Langston, C. (2017) Managing fluid and electrolyte disorders in kidney disease. *Veterinary Clinics of North America Small Animal Practice* 47, 471–490.

Libin, M.B., Weltman, J.G. and Prittie, J. (2020) A preliminary investigation into the association of chloride concentration on morbidity and mortality in hospitalized canine patients. *Veterinary Medicine (Auckland)* 11, 57–69.

Ostermann, M., Liu, K. and Kashani, K. (2019) Fluid management in acute kidney injury. *Chest* 156(3) 594–603.

Perner, A., Prowle, J., Joannidis, M. *et al.* (2017) Fluid management in acute kidney injury. *Intensive Care Medicine,* 43, 807-815.

Rein, J.L. and Coca, S.G. (2019) "I don't get no respect": the role of chloride in acute kidney injury. *American Journal of Physiology Renal Physiology* 316, F587–F605.

Self, W.H., Semler, M.W., Wanderer, J.P. *et al.* (2018) Balanced crystalloids versus saline in noncritically ill adults. *New England Journal of Medicine* 378, 819–828.

Young, P., Bailey, M., Beasley, R. *et al.* (2015) Effect of a buffered crystalloid solution vs saline on acute kidney injury among patients in the Intensive Care Unit: The SPLIT Randomized Clinical Trial. *Journal of the American Medical Association* 314, 1701–1710.

8v Anesthesia/Perioperative Fluid Considerations

JIWOONG HER

The Ohio State University, Columbus, Ohio, USA

Fluid therapy is routinely performed in patients undergoing anesthesia. The benefit of perioperative fluid therapy is the maintenance of end-organ perfusion and adequate tissue oxygen delivery by maintaining euvolemia. On the other hand, hypervolemia and excessive fluid administration are associated with increased morbidity and mortality (Fantoni and Shih, 2017). Potential adverse effects of positive fluid balance include pulmonary edema, decreased pulmonary function, prolonged ileus due to gut edema, increased risk of infection, electrolyte derangements, and dilutional coagulopathy. Therefore, an adequate amount of fluid administration before, during, and after anesthesia is of great importance.

The ideal rate of fluid administration during anesthesia continues to be a controversial topic. Decisions regarding the rate of fluid therapy depend on many factors. These include the patient's signalment, volume status, underlying disease, and the type of surgery or procedure. Previously, the traditional approach had been to administer fluid at 10–20 ml/kg/h. The rationale behind such supraphysiologic fluid rates was to offset hypotension, insensible fluid losses, poor tissue perfusion, anesthesia-induced vasodilation, and intraoperative blood loss (Fantoni and Shih, 2017). With recent evidence, most of these objectives are not actually achieved with perioperative fluids in that range. It has been shown that supraphysiologic fluid rate of lactated Ringer's solution at 10–30 ml/kg/h does not improve physiologic parameters (urine output, oxygen delivery to tissues, or arterial blood pressure) in healthy anesthetized dogs (Muir *et al.*, 2011). The reasons for this finding include the increased vascular capacitance due to venous relaxation caused by inhaled anesthetic agent, and rapid redistribution of infused fluid from the vascular space into peripheral or extravascular sites (Muir *et al.*, 2011). Intraoperative fluid therapy may even be harmful if administered excessively. The Confidential Inquiry into Perioperative Small Animal Fatalities identified perioperative fluid administration as an independent risk factor for increased mortality in cats (Brodbelt *et al.*, 2007). More recently, the American Animal Hospital Association published a guideline suggesting initial fluid rates at 5 ml/kg/h in dogs and 3 ml/kg/h in cats, although these rates were not based on any specific evidence (Davis *et al.*, 2013). Most importantly, not every patient responds to the given fluid rate equally, and so individualized goal-directed therapy should be used to determine the ideal fluid rate in perioperative settings. As such, these lower rates help to provide a starting point.

Balanced isotonic crystalloids (e.g., Normosol-R, Plasma-Lyte 148) are the most widely used for providing perioperative fluid therapy. Isotonic fluids are superior to hypotonic fluids for correction of hypovolemia due to fluid losses or anesthesia-induced vasodilation under anesthesia. Stress associated with general anesthesia and surgical pain leads to the stimulation of the neuroendocrine system, which is associated with decreased urine output, development of hyponatremia, and higher risk of fluid retention. The administration of a hypotonic solution (e.g., 0.45% NaCl) perioperatively may lead to hyponatremia, which is associated with poor outcomes in dogs and cats (Ueda, 2018).

Hypotension is one of the most common complications associated with general anesthesia, even in healthy dogs and cats (Davis *et al.*, 2013). As a first step, decreasing anesthetic depth may limit the hypotensive effect of anesthetic agents. If this is not successful in improving hemodynamic status, or the patient does not tolerate a lighter anesthetic plane, then fluid administration may be attempted. Potential guidelines for bolus fluid administration in these circumstances can be found in Table 8v.1.

DOI: 10.1079/9781789243406.0085

Table 8v.1. Suggested bolus dosages for hypotensive patient under anesthesia.

Type	Dosages
Isotonic crystalloid	10–15 ml/kg over 15–30 min (dog) 5–10 ml/kg over 15–30 min (cat)
Hydroxyethyl starch solutions	3–5 ml/kg over 15–30 min (dog) 2–3 ml/kg over 15–30 min (cat)
Fresh frozen plasma	3–5 ml/kg over 15–30 min (dog) 2–3 ml/kg over 15–30 min (cat)
7–7.5% Hypertonic saline	3–5 ml/kg over 5–10 min (do not exceed 1 ml/kg/min)
Packed red blood cells (for bleeding/anemic patient)	3–5 ml/kg over 15–30 min (dog) 2–3 ml/kg over 15–30 min (cat)
Fresh whole blood (for bleeding/anemic patient)	5–10 ml/kg over 15–30 min (dog) 4–6 ml/kg over 15–30 min (cat)

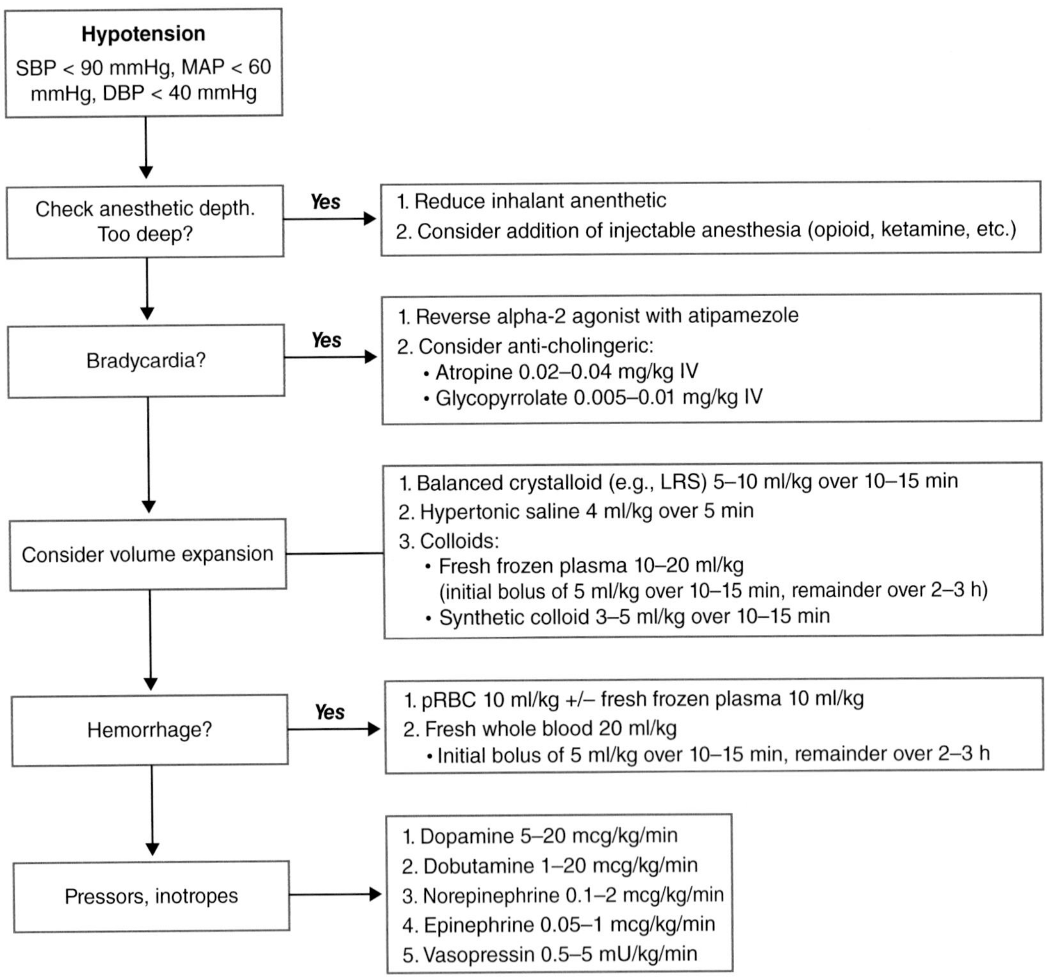

Fig. 8v.1. Suggested algorithm for addressing hypotension during anesthesia. (© The Ohio State University.) DBP, Doppler blood pressure; MAP, mean arterial blood pressure; SBP, systolic blood pressure.

The choice of crystalloid, colloid or blood product can be impacted by a number of different factors, including the reason for anesthesia, whether intra-operative blood loss has occurred, and patient co-morbidities (such as hypoproteinemia, cardiac disease, etc.). See Chapter 6i for more information.

Monitoring fluid resuscitation for patients under anesthesia can be challenging. For awake patients, fluid therapy is guided by hydration parameters, perfusion parameters, and other parameters such as blood pressure and urine output. While patients are under anesthesia, these parameters are altered by other factors such as surgical pain and physiological stress. In addition, analgesic and anesthetic drugs blunt sympathetic activity, thus reducing the ability of splanchnic circulation to mobilize blood into systemic circulation in response to absolute or relative hypovolemia. If fluid bolus is indicated to correct anesthesia-related hypotension, the adequacy of fluid therapy should be evaluated using hemodynamic indices to optimize the patient's volume status. Dynamic indices (e.g., pulse pressure variation, stroke volume variation, systolic pressure variation, and plethysmographic waveform variation) have been shown to be better guides for fluid responsiveness than static indices (e.g., central venous pressure, mean arterial pressure) (Fantoni and Shih, 2017). That being said, these dynamic assessments might not be available in many practice situations. It is also important to note that there is no single variable to precisely estimate intravascular volume status in patients under anesthesia. The most important part is to perform serial patient evaluations to optimize volume status. If the patient's response to a crystalloid bolus is inadequate, other options for volume expansion (e.g., administration of blood products or synthetic colloids), administering positive inotropes (such as dobutamine), or provision of vasopressors (such as norepinephrine) are indicated (Fig. 8v.1). Synthetic colloid should be used with caution, due to its adverse effects on renal function and coagulation (Holowaychuk, 2018).

Clinical Case 8v.1

A 1-year-old, 20 kg male neutered Labrador with a body condition score (BCS) 5/9 is presented to your clinic this afternoon for non-obstructive intestinal foreign body. On presentation, the patient is bright, alert, and responsive. He is estimated to be 5% dehydrated. It was elected to provide supportive care overnight and recheck abdominal radiographs tomorrow morning.

The rate of intravenous fluid overnight is determined by the following equation:

Volume of fluid required = fluid deficit + maintenance volume

Fluid deficit (20 kg × 0.05 × 1,000 ml = 1000 ml) over 18 h = 55 ml/h

Maintenance rate = 132 × (20 kg)0.75/24 h = 52 ml/h

Total 107 ml/h of isotonic crystalloid (e.g., Normosol-R, Plasma-Lyte 148)

Next morning, recheck radiographs show static foreign material with evidence of mechanical obstruction. The patient remained anorexic overnight but appeared to be normally hydrated. It is elected to place the patient under general anesthesia for foreign body removal. Therefore, the patient was placed on isotonic fluid at 100 ml/h (5 ml/kg/h) intraoperatively. During anesthesia, the patient developed mild hypotension. Initially the concentration of isoflurane was reduced from 1.5% to 1%; however, the patient became too light and had to be returned to 1.5%. It was decided to give a bolus of isotonic crystalloid (lactated Ringer's). He was given a fluid bolus at 10 ml/kg delivered over 20 min to which his blood pressure responded well. No further hypotension was noted, and the remainder of anesthesia was uneventful.

Clinical Case 8v.2

An 8-year-old 35 kg spayed female German Shepherd is presented to your clinic for sudden collapse. On initial vitals she is moderately tachycardic (150 bpm) with pale-pink mucous membranes and moderate pulse quality. She is found to have a Doppler blood pressure of 110 mm Hg. Based on diagnostics, the patient is found to have hemoabdomen secondary to solitary splenic mass. Peripheral packed cell volume and total solid on presentation are 35% and 4.2 g/dl, respectively. Exploratory laparotomy is elected for

Continued

Clinical Case 8v.2 Continued.

emergency splenectomy. With the concern for active bleeding and an acceptable blood pressure, it is decided not to administer any fluid boluses prior to surgery and initial fluid rate is determined as 5 ml/kg/h = 100 ml/h.

Once inhalant anesthetics are started, the patient's mean arterial blood pressure drops to 45 mm Hg. A significant amount of hemorrhagic effusion is noted on abdomen exploration. It is decided to give a bolus of isotonic crystalloid while preparing a transfusion of packed red blood cells. She is given Plasma-Lyte at 10 ml/kg (350 ml) delivered over 20 min, to which her blood pressure shows minimal improvement. A packed red blood cell transfusion is given following the fluid bolus. She is given a packed red blood cell bolus at 5 ml/kg (175 ml) delivered over 20 min, to which her blood pressure is normalized. Another 5 ml/kg of packed red blood cell is delivered over the next 1 h until the splenectomy is completed. No further hypotension or adverse reactions are noted, and the patient recovers uneventfully.

References

Brodbelt, D.C., Pfeiffer, D.U., Young, L.E. and Wood, J.L. (2007) Risk factors for anaesthetic-related death in cats: results from the confidential enquiry into perioperative small animal fatalities (CEPSAF). *British Journal of Anaesthesia* 99(5), 617–623.

Davis, H., Jensen, T., Johnson, A. *et al.* (2013) 2013 AAHA/AAFP fluid therapy guidelines for dogs and cats. *Journal of the American Animal Hospital Association* 49(3), 149–159.

Fantoni, D. and Shih, A.C. (2017) Perioperative fluid therapy. *Veterinary Clinics of North America: Small Animal Practice* 47(2), 423–434.

Holowaychuk, M.K. (2018) Colloid fluid therapy. In: Drobatz, K.J., Hopper, K., Rozanski, E. and Silverstein, D.C. (eds) *Textbook of Small Animal Emergency Medicine*. John Wiley & Sons, Hoboken, New Jersey, pp. 1097–1102.

Muir, W.W., Kijtawornrat, A., Ueyama, Y. *et al.* (2011) Effects of intravenous administration of lactated Ringer's solution on hematologic, serum biochemical, rheological, hemodynamic, and renal measurements in healthy isoflurane-anesthetized dogs. *Journal of the American Veterinary Medical Association* 239(5), 630–637.

Ueda, Y. (2018) Sodium and water balance. In: Drobatz, K.J., Hopper, K., Rozanski, E. and Silverstein, D.C. (eds) *Textbook of Small Animal Emergency Medicine*. John Wiley & Sons, Hoboken, New Jersey, pp. 690–699.

8vi Management of Hypernatremia and Hyponatremia

JULIEN GUILLAUMIN

Colorado State University, Fort Collins, Colorado, USA

Dysnatremic patients are considered challenging to manage, but the physiology behind both hyponatremia and hypernatremia is relatively straightforward. For the most part, measured changes in sodium are a function of changes in free water: **hyponatremia** from free water retention, and **hypernatremia** from water loss. What follows is an overview of causes for changes in sodium and how fluid therapy can be used to correct these abnormalities.

8vi.1 Hyponatremia

Hyponatremia is the most common sodium disturbance in small animals. It usually results from excess of free water secondary to antidiuretic hormone (ADH) secretion triggered by absolute hypovolemia or a decrease in effective circulating volume (see Box 8vi.1). Simply stated, in most circumstances the presence of hyponatremia means that there is too much water, not that there is too little sodium. Therefore, most often hyponatremia can be corrected by fixing the hypovolemia that caused it, with a fluid concentration that is close to the patient's sodium concentration. Overzealous use of 0.9% NaCl (which has the highest sodium concentration at 154 mEq/l) trying to "replace" sodium is a common mistake while managing hyponatremic patients and can be detrimental.

There are some circumstances when excessive ADH is released not in response to hypovolemia or changes in osmolality but, rather, triggered by other stimuli. This is referred to as the syndrome of inappropriate ADH secretion (SIADH) and can be another potential cause of hyponatremia. Discussion of SIADH is beyond the scope of this chapter, as treatment is geared toward identifying and addressing the underlying cause (such as intracranial disease, pneumonia, and opioids), as well as diuretic administration. Hyponatremia may also develop with severe hyperglycemia. This occurs because the excessive glucose pulls water into the vascular space, essentially diluting the sodium concentration (Box 8vi.1).

If acute (i.e., a few hours) plasma hyponatremia happens, an osmotic gradient will develop and water will shift into neurons, thereby increasing brain cell volume and creating severe acute brain edema. If a similar hyponatremia happens over several days, the neurons will promote an extracellular shift of electrolytes as well as idiogenic osmoles (i.e., osmolytes) to better match interstitial osmolality. This allows a more normal balance of water to exist and prevent the development of neuronal edema (although it does not correct brain hyperosmolality). This explains why chronic hyponatremia causes minimal clinical signs.

However, if the correction of chronic hyponatremia is too rapid, it can provoke osmotic water movement out of the cells and neuronal shrinkage. In addition to the immediate changes, rapid correction of hyponatremia (as well as rapid hypernatremia) may cause a delayed syndrome, called osmotic demyelination syndrome (ODS) or central pontine demyelination (CPD). This syndrome is characterized by irreversible neurological damage, including ataxia, paresis, dysphagia, or coma.

The goal of correction of chronic severe hyponatremia (or hypernatremia) is to limit changes in sodium to 0.5 mEq/l/h, or a maximum of 10–12 mEq/l/day. Acute hyponatremia can be corrected relatively quickly (1–2 mEq/l/h or quicker), if the clinician is sure the change is acute. Usually, there is no need to use a high-sodium-containing fluid. However, in the case reviewed below, we would use the sodium deficit calculation. After calculating the sodium deficit (in mEq), the goal would be to replace

DOI: 10.1079/9781789243406.0086

over a certain number of hours, at an average rate of 0.5 mEq/l/h. The rate will depend on the sodium content of the chosen fluid (see below). Usually, rechecks are needed every 6–8 h, to follow the progression of the correction of the hyponatremia.

8vi.2 Hypernatremia

Conversely, hypernatremia means "not enough water", either by removing free water (mostly by evaporation from skin or the respiratory system) or by adding sodium (e.g., following intravenous fluid therapy). Hypernatremia is most commonly caused by losing more water than sodium from gastrointestinal or renal losses. It can also be caused if the patient does not have access to water, or has a diminished/absent thirst mechanism. Loss of free water through osmotic diuresis or lack of ADH secretion/action is also common (central or nephrogenic diabetes insipidus). Much less common would be a gain in sodium from salt poisoning, hypertonic fluid administration or hyperaldosteronism. See Box 8vi.2 for a list of causes.

Similarly (although in the opposite direction) to what happens in chronic hyponatremia, chronic hypernatremia induces increased production of osmolytes to match the hyperosmolality, leading to normalization of neuronal volume. This explains why only acute hypernatremia leads to clinical signs. Clinical signs may arise in cases of acute normalization of chronic hypernatremia, when the rapid lowering of extracellular sodium may cause neuronal edema.

The treatment of chronic hypernatremia is relatively straightforward. Understanding and addressing the underlying cause is important, and is usually easily identified. Correction of hypernatremia (i.e., free water loss) is achieved by free water replacement. The rate for correction of hypernatremia is identical to the correction of hyponatremia, with a maximum of 12 mEq/l/day and goal of 0.5–1 mEq/l/h. The free water deficit calculation will be reviewed below, as well as the fluid type used to correct the free water loss.

Box 8vi.1. Selected causes of hyponatremia.

Hypovolemia
Gastrointestinal losses
Third-space losses
Severe burns
Hypoadrenocorticism
Diuretic administration
Hypervolemia
Liver disease
Congestive heart failure
Nephrotic syndrome
Advanced kidney disease
Hyperglycemia
Syndrome of inappropriate ADH secretion (SIADH)

Box 8vi.2. Selected causes of hypernatremia.

Pure water deficit	Sodium gain	Hypotonic fluid loss
No access to water	Salt toxicity	Gastrointestinal
Loss of thirst mechanism	Hypertonic fluid administration	Third-space loss
Diabetes insipidus	Hyperaldosteronism	Burns
• Central		Osmotic diuresis
• Nephrogenic		Post-obstructive diuresis
		Chronic kidney disease

Clinical Case 8vi.1. Hyponatremia

A 30 kg Labrador is presented to you with a 2–3-week history of weight loss, gastrointestinal signs, and polyuria/polydipsia. Upon diagnostics, you believe that the dog is suffering from chronic kidney disease and one of the main blood-work abnormalities is a serum sodium of 122 mmol/l. You are trying to create a fluid therapy, planning for the correction of the chronic hyponatremia.

First, one will have to assume that this hyponatremia is persistent despite (interstitial) rehydration with isotonic fluid. In hypovolemic patients, it is not uncommon that the ADH secretion is triggered and therefore some degree of hyponatremia can be due to hypovolemia and appropriate ADH trigger.

What fluid type?

As usual, fluid therapy planning consists of choosing the fluid type, then the fluid volume, and then the time-frame of replacement. Also important in this case is that the fluid volume depends on the fluid type chosen. In this case, 0.9% NaCl is selected that has a sodium concentration of 154 mmol/l.

How much volume?

The volume depends on the fluid type, because of the impact of the sodium content of the fluid. There are various ways to address the calculation of the volume to be given. One of them is to calculate the sodium deficit using the following formula:

Sodium deficit (in mmol)

= 0.6 × BW (kg) × (Normal Na – Patient Na)

= 0.6 × 30 × (145–122) for this specific patient

= 414 mmol

This formula provides an amount of sodium to be provided, in mEq. The next step is knowing the sodium content of the fluid you are using. As 0.9% NaCl, the fluid we chose, has sodium at 154 mmol/l, providing 414 mmol of sodium requires 2.7 l, or 2700 ml, of 0.9% NaCl.

How fast?

As previously stated for hypernatremia, the rate of increased sodium should be between 0.5 and 1 mmol/l/h, so 23–46 h to raise sodium from 122 mmol/l to 145 mmol/l. If 36 h is chosen, then 0.9% NaCl would be given at the rate of 75 ml/h, which is 2700 ml divided by 36 h.

Note: One formula can be used to calculate the rate of infusion, integrating the various steps seen above:

Rate of infusion (in ml/h)

= [0.6 × BW_{kg} × (normal Na – patient Na) × 1000] / (fluid Na content × timeframe of replacement (h)

= [0.6 × 30 × (145–122) × 1000]/(154 × 36)

= 414000/5580

= 74ml / h

Clinical Case 8vi.2. Hypernatremia

A 5-year-old, 5 kg domestic shorthair cat is hospitalized at your veterinary clinic for fever of unknown origin. The sodium at admission is 145 mmol/l and 3 days later the serum sodium level is rechecked at 175 mmol/l. The cat does not present any physical examination signs of extracellular dehydration and does not appear to be in shock.

The cat has documented hypernatremia, and its sodium goes up 30 mmol/l in 3 days. The assumption is that the pet had free water loss caused by the fever. As we indicated in this chapter, being hypernatremic means that the cat is missing free water. As usual, we would divide our fluid therapy planning into three parts, first choosing the fluid type, then choosing the fluid volume, and finally the time-frame for the fluid replacement.

What fluid type?

As our first example, we would choose dextrose 5% in water (D5W) as our replacement fluid. Because it contains only water after the dextrose has been metabolized, D5W is a hypotonic iso-osmolar fluid.

How much volume?

We will then calculate the free water deficit (FWD) using the following formula:

FWD

= 0.6 × BW_{kg} × [(current sodium value) / normal sodium value −1]

= 0.6 × 5 × [(175 / 145) – 1)]for this specific patient

= 0.620l

= 620ml

Remember that, as the body weight is in kilograms, the final volume is in liters.

Continued

Clinical Case 8vi.2. Continued.

How fast?

For this patient, there is a documented time-frame of 3 days, and we should replace the volume deficit in order to drop the sodium from 175 mmol/l to 145 mmol/l at a rate of 0.5–1 mmol/l/h. Therefore, a replacement strategy would be to replace the deficit over 30–60 h. For this case example, the 620 ml of free water deficit will be replaced over 48 h, which ends up being 13 ml/h for 48 h.

Note: If the choice of fluid type is 0.45% NaCl, then the volume deficit is the same (620 ml). However, as 0.45% contains roughly 50% water (relative normal osmolality), 1 ml of 0.45% NaCl only contains 0.5 ml of "pure water". Replacing a volume deficit of 620 ml of water will therefore require 1240 ml of 0.45% NaCl. This volume can be given over the same time-frame of 48 h, so 26 ml/h.

8vii Approach to Fluid Therapy in Patients with Hypoproteinemia

JULIEN GUILLAUMIN

Colorado State University, Fort Collins, Colorado, USA

Disorders such as protein-losing nephropathy, protein-losing enteropathy, malabsorptive disorders, and liver failure can lead to moderate to severe hypoproteinemia. Dogs and cats with hypoproteinemia are often challenging to manage clinically, depending on the severity of the hypoproteinemia, and the associated clinical signs. Albumin, globulins, and other proteins contribute to a colloid osmotic pressure (COP), also known as oncotic pressure, with albumin itself contributing 70–80% of COP. Therefore, hypoproteinemia, especially hypoalbuminemia, is usually associated with a decreased oncotic pressure. In return, this affects the movement of fluid out of the vascular space. Even with the new understanding of the Starling forces, decreases in oncotic pressure will lead to the tendency of fluid to leave the intravascular compartment toward the interstitial fluid compartment, and may lead to edema (see Chapter 2).

Hypoproteinemia can lead to leakage of fluid into third spaces (i.e., neither intracellular nor extracellular) such as pleural or abdominal effusion (typically characterized as a pure transudate with low protein and low cellularity). This results in decreased plasma volume, leading to hypovolemia, as well as an increase in interstitial fluid water, or edema.

To build a fluid therapy plan for a hypoproteinemic dog or cat, we would start with choosing the right fluid. It stands to reason that choosing a fluid type that is more likely to remain within the vascular compartment makes the most sense, with the goal of limiting the extravasation of fluid into the interstitial fluid compartment. Fluid options include hypotonic or isotonic crystalloids, and natural or synthetic colloids. As **hypotonic fluids** are usually used for free-water replacement in patients with hypernatremia, and will distribute across the total body water, they are not a suitable option. **Isotonic fluids**, a common fixture in clinical practice, may not be ideal for these patients. Indeed, 75% of the volume given would go into the interstitium even if the oncotic pressure was normal. Given that it is likely to be lower in these patients, an even greater portion will extravasate into the intersitium. Therefore, it is important to limit the use of isotonic crystalloids in these patients. In the circumstances of dehydration and hypoproteinemia, the rate of replacement for the calculated dehydration should be slower, maybe over 24 h or more, compared with a similar patient with a normal albumin level and oncotic pressure.

Therefore, when fluid administration is needed for hypoproteinemic patients, the most appropriate fluid type is colloids. Colloids are more likely to remain within the vasculature space, and the rate of transfer across the intersitium is very slow. **Synthetic colloids** are hyperoncotic, meaning that their oncotic pressures are higher than the plasma. However, synthetic molecules can be trapped in the endothelial surface layer if the endothelium glycocalyx is disrupted, and actually encourage movement into the interstitium (Kang and Yoo, 2019). Thus, they may not be ideal for hypoalbuminemic patients, depending on the health status of the endothelial glycocalyx and the endothelial cells. Some synthetic colloids have been associated with increased risks of kidney injury in people, although the evidence in veterinary medicine is inconsistent (Adamik and Yozova, 2021; Montealegre and Lyons, 2021). Other side effects include a dose-dependent platelet dysfunction. Note that synthetic colloids such as hydroxethyl starches are banned in some countries, especially in Europe, and gelatins (another synthetic colloid) may be used in replacement. See Chapter 4i for additional information regarding synthetic colloids.

DOI: 10.1079/9781789243406.0087

With the concerns regarding the use of synthetic colloids, **natural colloids** (when available) are the most appropriate fluid for administration to the hypoproteinemic dog and cat. Natural colloids, in the form of concentrated canine albumin, fresh frozen plasma (FFP), or cryo-poor plasma (CPP), are a source of albumin and oncotic pressure. Concentrated canine albumin can be diluted to concentrations ranging from 5% to 16% solution, resulting in an albumin level of 5 g/dl (50 mg/ml) to 16 g/dl (160 mg/ml). A 5% albumin solution is roughly iso-oncotic to the plasma, whereas a 16% solution is hyperoncotic. Fresh frozen plasma contains approximately 2.9 g/dl (29 mg/ml) and has an oncotic pressure of approximately 12.7 mm Hg. Therefore, it is mildly hypo-oncotic compared with plasma. The major drawbacks of natural colloids are price and availability. For an assortment of reasons, the use of human albumin is not recommended (see Chapter 4ii).

If a synthetic colloid is chosen, particularly in the circumstance that natural colloid is not available, the dose depends on the synthetic colloid used. For acute volume expansion in resuscitation, the dose is typically 3–5 ml/kg. For ongoing administration as a constant rate infusion (CRI), dosing can range from 20–50 ml/kg/day, which equates to 1–2 ml/kg/h. If used as a CRI, particular caution should be exercised in patients with known underlying kidney disease.

If a natural colloid such as FFP is used, dosing and rate will depend on goals of administration. If there is concern for hypovolemic shock, then a resuscitative dose of 3–5 ml/kg can be given over 15–30 min. The patient is then reassessed to determine if additional doses are needed. For ongoing administration to address hypoalbuminemia and hypoproteinemia there is no set dose for "maintenance" rate of FFP or CPP. Some clinicians will use a "standard" dose similar to synthetic colloids, such as 1–2 ml/kg/h or 20–50 ml/kg/day. However, others may use a "standard" dose of FFP aimed at addressing coagulopathy, which is 20 ml/kg/day, and provided as a CRI. Along these lines, it has been demonstrated that CPP at 0.8 ml/kg/h was associated with a rise of albumin from 1.5 g/dl to 2.1 g/dl in a retrospective study of ten critically ill hypoalbuminemic dogs (Culler *et al.*, 2019).

A fixed dose of **plasma** is recommended, as formula-driven dosing depends on the formula used. For example, the commonly used formula to calculate the "albumin deficit" (10 × desired albumin increase × weight (kg) × 0.3) comes from human literature related to total parenteral nutrition (Hardin *et al.*, 1986). The commonly quoted "20 ml/kg of FFP will raise albumin by 0.5 g/dl" is from unreferenced literature and contradicts the albumin deficit formula (which would suggest closer to 40 ml/kg is needed) (Mazzaferro *et al.*, 2002). In the absence of evidence-based guidelines, it is reasonable to consider a fixed dose in the range of 20–40 ml/kg/day. This works out as approximately 1–2 ml/kg/h, a rate commonly used for supporting albumin levels in critically ill dogs, and this is similar to the recommended dose of albumin in people (around 0.7–1 g/kg/day).

Clinical Case 8vii.1

Lumiere is a 6-year-old, 15.3 kg castrated male French Bulldog that developed generalized edema after a routine spinal surgery. His pre-anesthesia workup showed the following data:

Biochemistry profile	
BUN	96 mg/dl
Creatinine	2.2 mg/dl
Na	148 mmol/l
Albumin	2.9 g/dl
Globulin	2.2 g/dl
Complete blood count	
Hematocrit	53%
Platelet count	177 × 10^9/l
White blood cell count	14.2 × 10^9/l
Urinalysis	
SpG	1.025
Protein	3+
UPC	22.1

His spinal surgery was routine, but he received a large amount of isotonic crystalloid during the pre- and post-anesthesia time in order to treat his kidney values, which were presumed to be pre-renal at that time. By the day following surgery he has started to develop generalized edema and an increase in respiratory effort.

As the patient is reassessed, his rectal temperature is 100.7°F (38.2°C), his heart rate is 90 bpm and his respiratory rate is 60 rpm with mild dyspnea. His weight has increased to 16.8 kg. He has profound

Continued

Clinical Case 8vii.1. Continued.

generalized pitting edema with no signs of hypovolemic shock. He has decreased lung sounds ventrally and bilaterally and an abdominal fluid wave. His repeat diagnostic results are:

Biochemistry profile	
BUN	69 mg/dl
Creatinine	1.5 mg/dl
Na	137 mmol/l
Albumin	1.5 g/dl
Globulin	1.7 g/dl
Complete blood count	
Hematocrit	28%
Platelet count	234×10^9/l
White blood cell count	34.6×10^9/l
Point-of-care ultrasound	
Abdominal	Positive for free peritoneal fluid
Thoracic	Positive for pleural and pericardial free fluid

Based on physical examination findings and the presence of pleural effusion, you elect to perform a diagnostic and therapeutic thoracocentesis, which yields 155 ml of clear fluid that you identify as a transudate. Based on the information gathered during your history and physical examination, your working diagnosis is some type of glomerular disease resulting in hypoproteinemia and decreased renal function exacerbated by anesthesia. Further, intravenous fluid therapy with isotonic crystalloid may have disrupted the delicate balance secondary to Starling's forces and endothelial glycocalyx. You now must design a fluid therapy plan for this patient.

As is the case with any fluid therapy plan, the first step is deciding what type of fluid to use. The options for this patient would be hypotonic or isotonic crystalloids, or natural or synthetic colloids. For the reasons discussed above, use of fresh frozen plasma would be ideal in this patient.

With this in mind, the isotonic crystalloid he has been receiving is stopped, as it obviously disrupted the delicate equilibrium of the endothelium. Using a target of FFP at 1–2 ml/kg/h, Lumiere is started on FFP at 20 ml/h. This volume of FFP corresponds to roughly two 250 ml units of FFP per day, which is economically feasible. When using FFP as a CRI, it is important to make sure that plasma is only at room temperature for 4–6 h, otherwise the risk of contamination may increase (Brunskill *et al.*, 2012). This can be accomplished by aseptically separating the needed volume (in this case 80–120 ml to provide 4–6 h of infusion at 20 ml/h) and keeping the rest of the volume in the refrigerator until needed.

Lumiere also receives a low dose of furosemide (1 mg/kg) in order to help mobilize some of the interstitial fluid by promoting renal sodium and water loss. The resulting decrease in hydrostatic pressure thereby modifies Starling forces to lessen tissue and cavitary fluid accumulation.

Over the next few days, Lumiere is able to lose the fluids he had accumulated, and his edema drastically improves. He is discharged after 5 days of hospitalization at 15.5 kg.

References

Adamik, K.N. and Yozova, I.D. (2021) Colloids yes or no? – a “Gretchen question” answered. *Frontiers in Veterinary Science* 8, 624049.

Brunskill, S., Thomas, S., Whitmore, E. *et al.* (2012) What is the maximum time that a unit of red blood cells can be safely left out of controlled temperature storage? *Transfusion Medicine Reviews* 26(3), 209–223.

Culler, C.A., Balakrishnan, A., Yaxley, P.E. and Guillaumin, J. (2019) Clinical use of cryopoor plasma continuous rate infusion in critically ill, hypoalbuminemic dogs. *Journal of Veterinary Emergency and Critical Care* 29(3), 314–320.

Hardin, T.C., Page, C.P. and Schwesinger, W.H. (1986) Rapid replacement of serum albumin in patients receiving total parenteral nutrition. *Surgery, Gynecology, and Obstetrics* 163(4), 359–362.

Kang, D. and Yoo, K.Y. (2019) Fluid management in perioperative and critically ill patients. *Acute Critical Care* 34(4), 235–245.

Mazzaferro, E., Rudloff, E. and Kirby, R. (2002) Role of albumin in the veterinary critically ill patient. *Journal of Veterinary Emergency and Critical Care* 12(2), 113–124.

Montealegre, F. and Lyons, B.M. (2021) Fluid therapy in dogs and cats with sepsis. *Frontiers in Veterinary Science* 8, 622127.

8viii Special Considerations in Neonates/Pediatrics

PAGE YAXLEY

The Ohio State University, Columbus, Ohio, USA

Dogs and cats are considered **pediatric** in the first 4–6 months of life (McMichael and Duhpa, 2000a; Macintire, 2008; Lee and Cohn, 2017). This pediatric period can be further subcategorized into the **neonatal stage** (birth to 2 weeks of life), the **infant stage** (2–6 weeks of life), and the **juvenile stage** (6–12 weeks of life) (McMichael and Duhpa, 2000a; Macintire, 2008; Lee and Cohn, 2017). While most puppies and kittens are weaned by 8 weeks of life, they are still considered pediatric until 4–6 months of life. The medical care for pediatric patients can be challenging, due to their relative size, unique physiology, and limit for compensatory mechanisms, making them susceptible to rapid onset of critical illness. The first weeks of a pediatric patient's life represent a high-risk period of abnormal developmental events, and extrinsic insults (Lawler, 2008). For these reasons, pediatric patients may present to the veterinarian dehydrated or in shock. Commonly associated predisposing conditions for critical illness are listed in Table 8viii.1. Fluid therapy is often required for these pediatric patients, but methods to identify clinical signs and to provide fluids vary, given the stage of life and severity of underlying condition (Macintire, 2008; Munnich and Kuchenmeister, 2014).

8viii.1 Pediatric Physiology

Fluid requirements in pediatric patients are significantly different from the adult counterpart, due to alterations in fluid compartments and unique physiology. Neonates have higher **extracellular fluid** on a volume per kilogram basis (80% of body weight, compared with 60% in adult animals) (McMichael and Duhpa, 2000a; Lawler, 2008; Macintire, 2008; Lee and Cohn, 2017). Pediatric patients have a higher **metabolic demand**, resulting in an increased use of water. This accelerated water turnover can result in rapid onset of dehydration (Poffenberger *et al.*, 1990). A larger body surface area to volume ratio as well as increased skin permeability results in a larger inherent loss (Lawler, 2008; Macintire, 2008; Lee and Cohn, 2017). Increased ambient temperature can heighten the evaporative losses through the skin, and result in dehydration and subsequent constipation (Gunn-Moore, 2006; Lawler, 2008, Munnich and Kuchenmeister, 2014).

Pediatrics are unable to respond adequately to **hypovolemia**, due to their unique cardiovascular physiology. In the adult patient, cardiac output is the product of heart rate and stroke volume. Adaptations to combat hypovolemia include compensatory mechanisms of the sympathetic nervous system to increase catecholamine release, thereby increasing cardiac output. Likewise, stimulation of renin–angiotensin–aldosterone system and release of anti-diuretic hormone aid in fluid retention and vasoconstriction, increasing stroke volume to restore cardiac output. Pediatric patients largely lack these compensatory mechanisms. Decreased sympathetic innervation of the myocardium (in puppies) and decreased contractile elements in fetal cardiac muscle result in an inability to increase cardiac output through increased heart rate (Mace and Levy, 1983; McMichael and Dhupa, 2000b; Lee and Cohn, 2017).

Since **renal function** is not mature at birth, pediatrics lose water through urine. The normal urine specific gravity in the neonate ranges from 1.006 to 1.071 (Crawford, 1995; Munnich and Kuchenmeister, 2014). Pediatric patients have a higher glomerular filtration rate, higher daily urine output, higher free water reabsorption, and lower daily protein excretion and fractional excretion of phosphorus (Laroute *et al.*, 2005). Additionally, neonates may

DOI: 10.1079/9781789243406.0088

Table 8viii.1. Age-related predisposing conditions for the development of critical illness.

Neonatal	Infant	Juvenile
Dystocia Hypoxia induced Hypoperfusion Failure of passive transfer Inadequate suckle Agalactia, hypoglycemia Hypothermia Poor mothering Separation from dam Congenital deficits Husbandry-related issue Trauma Fading syndrome Sepsis	Hypoglycemia Parasitism (internal or external) Trauma Overfeeding Improper nutrition Diarrhea	Infectious diseases • Viral • Bacterial

have decreased autoregulation of renal blood flow and therefore may not be able to respond to rapid sodium and water fluctuations (Kleinman and Lubbe, 1972; Kleinman and Reuter, 1974; Jose *et al.*, 1975; Fettman and Allen; 1991; Lee and Cohn, 2017). Controversy remains as to when pediatric patients develop the ability to concentrate their urine. Most believe that pediatrics gain concentrating ability (>1.030) around 8 weeks of age, but reports exist from as young as 4 weeks and as old as 12 weeks (Poffenberger *et al.*, 1990; Faulks and Lane, 2003; Macintire, 2008; Lee and Cohn, 2017).

8viii.2 Assessment of the Sick Neonate

Dehydration (interstitial and intracellular fluid loss) and **hypovolemia** (intravascular volume loss) can occur separately, or both be present in a single patient. Many reasons can cause dehydration in the pediatric patient, most of which are associated with the development of diarrhea (Macintire, 2008). Severe dehydration leads to hypovolemia as fluid is removed from the intravascular space to replenish the other fluid compartments. Due to their higher body water needs, these processes can rapidly progress, resulting in life-threatening illness.

Methods of hydration assessment commonly used in the adult patient do not carry over to the pediatric patient. As previously stated, urine concentration and presence of tachycardia will not be reliable. Mucous membrane color may be a reliable assessment for perfusion, but moisture content of the mucous membranes is difficult to assess in the tiny mouth, along with the presence of milk and constant suckling. Capillary refill time, also difficult to assess based on mouth size, is a late manifestation of severe dehydration and is not reliable (Macintire, 2008). Assessment of enophthalmos or sunken globes is not possible, as neonatal dogs and cats do not open their eyes until 2 weeks of age. The presence of loose skin makes skin turgor also unreliable, although some have suggested the skin on the ventral abdomen to be a potential source of assessment (Macintire, 2008) (Fig. 8viii.1). Hypovolemia is similarly difficult to assess, as pulse quality and jugular venous distensibility are often undeterminable (Lee and Cohn, 2017). Reliable clinical signs for assessment of hypovolemia, sepsis, and shock include bradycardia, pallor, decreased urine output, cold extremities and limp body tone, reluctance to suckle, or distress vocalization (Lawler, 2008; Macintire, 2008). The veterinarian should determine whether the patient has dehydration, hypovolemia, or both, and should receive fluid therapy consistent with the severity of disease (Macintire, 2008).

8viii.3 Fluid Type

Isotonic crystalloid replacement fluids resembling the extracellular fluid compartment can be safely administered to the pediatric patient (Macintire, 2008; Lee and Cohn, 2017). Previously there has been discrepancy as to whether or not to avoid lactate-containing fluids, due to the pediatric patient less than 6 weeks of age being unable to metabolically convert lactate to bicarbonate (Hoskins, 1995; Lee and Cohn, 2017). Others believe that lactate is utilized as an energy source in the neonate brain, and therefore lactate-containing fluids may actually be preferred (McMichael, 2005).

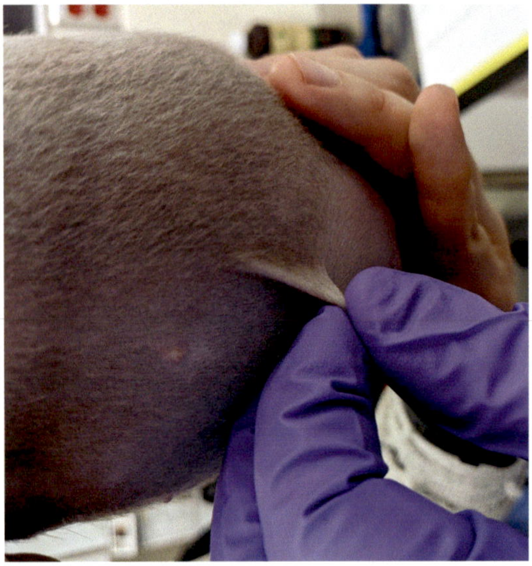

Fig. 8viii.1. Example of testing skin tent on the ventral abdomen of a puppy. (Image courtesy of Edward Cooper.)

Colloids may also be considered, when crystalloids fail, and in the presence of hypoalbuminemia. **Hypoalbuminemia** is one of three major biochemical changes of the failing neonate, in addition to hypoglycemia and hypovolemia (Lawler, 2008). Colloids, larger molecular weight fluid solutions, remain in the intravascular space longer and therefore may be attractive for both resuscitation and treatment of hypoalbuminemia (Lee and Cohn, 2017). Colloids can be either synthetic or natural. **Synthetic colloids** have been associated with risks including coagulopathy and acute kidney injury in the adult patient, but the effect on the pediatric patient remains undetermined. Synthetic colloids may be considered to target volume expansion. **Natural colloids** (albumin-containing fluids) may provide a viable source of albumin and globulins in small patients as compared with larger patients and have the added benefit of being able to be delivered through multiple routes of administration (Lee and Cohn, 2017).

Regardless of fluid type, all fluids should be warmed, as neonates are prone to **hypothermia**. They produce body heat through thermogenesis by catecholamine release and brown fat tissue metabolism up to day 6 postpartum (Munnich and Kuchenmeister, 2014). This process requires energy, contributing also to their propensity for hypoglycemia (Munnich and Kuchenmeister, 2014). Hypothermia can result in bradycardia and ileus and therefore should be avoided. Body temperature in the first 2 weeks of life is normally 95–99°F (35–37.2°C), 97–100°F (36.1–37.8°C) from day 14 to 28, and normal adult body temperature at 4 weeks of age (Lawler, 2008). Fluids run at slow rates through fluid lines cool rapidly, therefore it is necessary to take into account the fluid tubing as well as the bag or syringe (Lee and Cohn, 2017).

8viii.4 Route of Administration

The route of administration of fluids is dependent upon severity of illness, size of patient, technical skill, type of fluid being administered, and the susceptibility of the patient to bacterial insult (Lawler, 2008; Macintire, 2008; Lee and Cohn, 2017).

Oral administration is the preferred method for euvolemic, normothermic, normoglycemic, mildly dehydrated but stable, non-vomiting pediatric patients. Oral administration is the slowest means of replacement, and therefore is not a consideration for the sicker patient. In addition, hypothermic and/or patients in shock will have significantly decreased gastrointestinal absorption. Colostrum, milk replacer, dextrose, balanced electrolytes, and water can be administered via this route (Lawler, 2008; Macintire, 2008; Lee and Cohn, 2017). If the patient has a suckle response, fluid can be delivered through a nippled bottle, syringe or eyedropper (Macintire, 2008). This induces the least stress in the neonatal patient. The nipple hole can be created in the bottle with a sterilized needle large enough for liquid to bead when the bottle is inverted. If no suckle response is present, tube feeding can be performed. A 5 to 8 French feeding tube can be measured from the nose to last rib, marked and lubricated (Macintire, 2008). It is recommended to err on the side of a larger-bore tube, as smaller tubes can curl in the esophagus and result in aspiration (Lawler, 2008). The tube is passed through the left side of the mouth until the mark is reached. Neonates do not possess a gag response until day 10, therefore it is recommended to instill a small volume of sterile warmed water and check for nasal discharge. If no discharge is present, the patient can be administered fluid or nutrition. The tube should be kinked before removal (Macintire, 2008).

Subcutaneous fluid administration is the most commonly utilized parenteral route (Lawler, 2008). Subcutaneous administration is good for the euvolemic patient with mild dehydration, as the rate of absorption is slow (Lee and Cohn, 2017). Fluids can be warmed, and easily placed in multiple locations in the subcutaneous space (Macintire, 2008; Lee and Cohn, 2017). Daily maintenance dosages of isotonic fluid therapy can be divided and delivered subcutaneously over the day to reduce risk of overhydration (Macintire, 2008). Care should be taken not to provide dextrose supplementation subcutaneously, as this results in hypertonicity and drives fluid into the subcutaneous space.

Intraperitoneal fluid administration is another consideration for fluid replacement in the normovolemic neonatal patient. Once again, care to warm fluids is important to prevent hypothermia. Intraperitoneal fluid administration, performed through aseptic techniques, offers a technically easy, but slow rate of fluid absorption. Isotonic crystalloids, colostrum, and blood products can be administered through this route (Macintire, 2008; Lee and Cohn, 2017). Given that red blood cells are not absorbed for 48–72 h, life-threatening anemias should not be treated by this route. Intraperitoneal administration can induce some patient discomfort and repeated delivery through the peritoneal space is discouraged, due to increased risk of infection (Macintire, 2008; Lee and Cohn, 2017).

For severely dehydrated or hypovolemic patients, the preferred method of administration is **intravenous** or **intraosseous.** Access to the intramedullary canal with an 18–22-gauge needle can provide a reliable route of delivery for rapid administration of fluids and blood products (and medications) to a patient in shock. Performed using aseptic technique, the bone marrow sinusoid can be accessed through the greater tubercle of the humerus, trochanteric fossa of the femur, the tibial tuberosity or the ilial wing (Fig. 8viii.2). The needle is threaded down the canal and can be secured in place with suture or tape (Macintire, 2008; Lee and Cohn, 2017). Limiting factors for intraosseous placement include size of medullary canal, technical expertise, damage to the sciatic nerve, bone or cartilage, extravasation at the site, or osteomyelitis (Lawler, 2008; Munnich and Kuchenmeister, 2014). However, intraosseous placement remains a life-saving vascular access option for the neonatal patient.

Intravenous catheter placement can also provide vascular access to a pediatric patient. Using a 22–27-gauge catheter, the cephalic or jugular vein can be accessed using aseptic techniques. Cephalic catheters often require a brace (such as a tongue depressor) to prevent dislodgement. A padded neck wrap is generally placed to protect a jugular catheter (Fig. 8viii.3). Heparin flush should be avoided as it can perpetuate coagulopathy; instead, judicious use of saline is utilized to flush catheters (Lee and Cohn, 2017).

8viii.5 Fluid Dosages

Fluid dosages vary by the type of fluid, goal, and the route of administration (Lee and Cohn, 2017). For small patients, syringe pumps or volume infusers provide increased safety over a fluid pump or drip

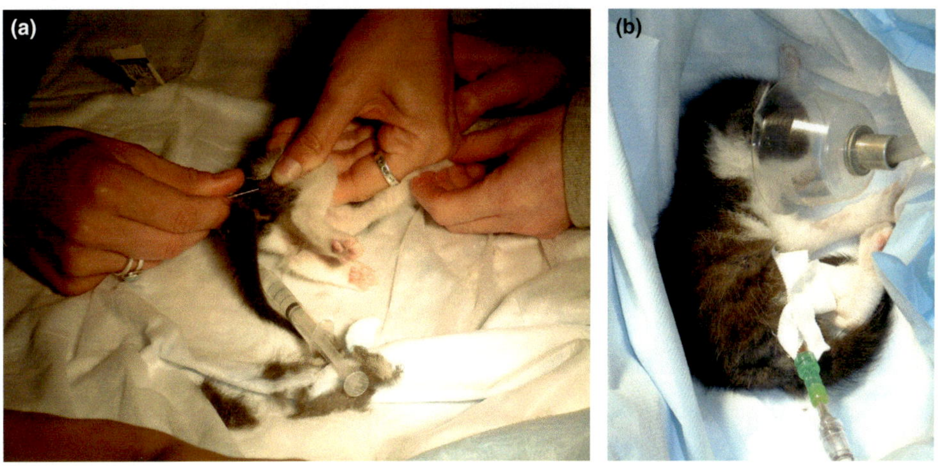

Fig. 8viii.2. (a) Placement of a 22-gauge needle into the trochanteric fossa of a pediatric kitten for intraosseous access. **(b)** Intraosseous needle with injection cap and secured with tape. (Figures courtesy of A. Brown.)

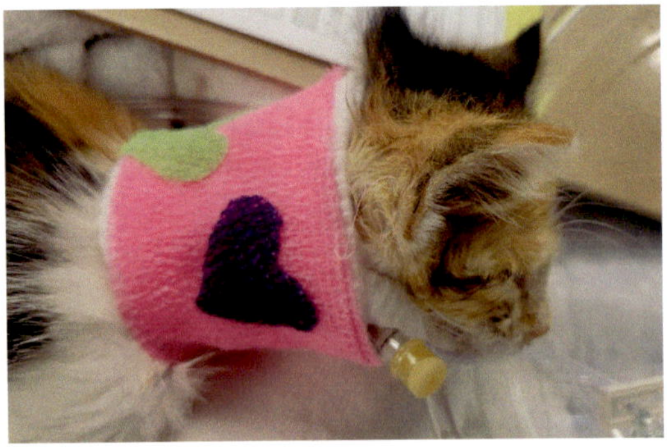

Fig. 8viii.3. Example of a kitten with a jugular catheter and neck wrap.

set alone (Lee and Cohn, 2017). The most accepted pediatric **maintenance fluid doses** for isotonic crystalloid fluid therapy are 80–120 ml/kg/day in the dog and 60–80 ml/kg/day in the cat. Maintenance rates are reduced to adult doses at 4–6 months of age (or the end of the pediatric period) (Macintire, 2008; Lee and Cohn, 2017). Others have proposed higher pediatric maintenance doses for crystalloid therapy, up to 180 ml/kg/day in dogs (Munnich and Kuchenmeister, 2014).

Resuscitation dosage for the hypovolemic pediatric patient with isotonic crystalloids is 3–4 ml/100 g body weight for dogs (30–40 ml/kg), and 2–3 ml/100 g of body weight for cats (20–30 ml/kg), administered intravenously or intraosseously over 10 min. In practice, the author prefers delivering shock doses over 20–30 min. Estimating and replacing dehydration is much more difficult in the pediatric patient for reasons previously stated. Crystalloid dosing to correct dehydration may be adjusted to 60–180 ml/kg/day with continuous monitoring and reassessment (Lawler, 2008). See Clinical Cases 8viii.1 and 8viii.2.

8viii.6 Monitoring

Following resuscitation or rehydration, the pediatric patient should be closely monitored, as reoccurrence is common (Lawler, 2008). Patient weights should be tracked daily as well as the mucous membrane color. Similarly, the dam's milk production should be monitored, and the patient should remain in appropriate ambient temperature for their age. Separation of the litter, hyperventilation, increased rectal temperature, increased skin temperature, and distress vocalization may signify too warm an ambient temperature.

Overhydration should be avoided. Too aggressive resuscitation or rehydration may result in cardiac overload, pulmonary edema, and intracranial hemorrhage (Lawler, 2008). Clinical signs associated with overhydration are subtle and include serous nasal discharge, chemosis, tachypnea or altered breathing effort, restlessness, cough, tachycardia, ascites, crackles, or polyuria (Lee and Cohn, 2017).

8viii.7 Discontinuation of Fluid Therapy

Once a pediatric patient is euhydrated and normovolemic, a slow weaning process can begin. Vigilance for recurrence of fluid loss should be maintained. If deemed appropriate the patient can be transitioned from a more aggressive fluid route (such as IV) to oral administration. If the patient tolerates this change, then the fluids can be weaned over a period of 2–4 days (Lee and Cohn, 2017).

8viii.8 Nutritional Considerations

Neonates can become dehydrated and subsequently hypovolemic if they do not have adequate nutrition. The **energy requirement** for neonates is 20-26 kcal/100 g body weight daily, delivered in multiple feedings (Lawler, 2008). All food or fluid fed should be warmed and delivered slowly. Milk replacement can be diluted 1:2 with a balanced electrolyte solution if diarrhea develops, to prevent dehydration (Macintire, 2008). The **stomach capacity** for a neonate is 40–50 ml/kg and care should be taken to not exceed or fill to capacity (Lawler, 2008; Macintire, 2008; Lee and Cohn, 2017). General recommendations are to feed approximately 10 ml every 2–4 h in puppies, and 5 ml every 2–4 h in kittens. Significant complications can result, including nasal discharge, regurgitation, abdominal distension and discomfort, and diarrhea, creating an unbalanced gastrointestinal flora, which can lead to sepsis. Box 8viii.1 gives an example of nutritional planning for a 500 g neonatal puppy.

8viii.9 Hypoglycemia and Hypokalemia

Pediatric patients are less metabolically able to generate glucose and have a much higher requirement compared with the adult patient. Periparturient complications, including placental insufficiency, prematurity, hypoxia, hypogalactia or agalactia, may increase the risk for hypoglycemic crisis (Lawler,

Clinical Case 8viii.1

A 7-day-old 300 g terrier puppy is presented to the hospital for failure to thrive. The puppy has a limp body condition and has a heart rate of 70 bpm and temperature of 96°F (35.6°C). The puppy was last normal 12 h ago and has developed mild mucoid diarrhea and has not been nursing. The puppy is normoglycemic.

The patient is identified as being hypovolemic and an intraosseous catheter is placed. To stabilize the patient, a bolus dose of warmed isotonic crystalloid fluids is prepared:

300 g × (4 ml /100g) = 12 ml bolus over 15–20 min

After the bolus, the patient's heart rate normalizes and the patient becomes more active.

A maintenance fluid rate is calculated:

300 g × (1kg /1000 g) × (80–120 ml)/(kg/day) × (1 day/24 h) = 1–1.5 ml/ h

Clinical Case 8viii.2

A 14-day-old 900 g puppy presents to the hospital for being slightly weaker and smaller than the rest of his littermates. The puppy has good muscle tone, normal heart rate and temperature. You believe the puppy to be mildly dehydrated based on the history and skin turgor on his ventral abdomen. You elect to give the puppy subcutaneous fluids. A daily maintenance rate is calculated:

900 g × (1kg/ 1000 g) × (80 –120 ml) / (kg/day) = 72 – 108 ml/day

You instruct the owner to give 25 ml SQ every 6 h for the next 24 h.

Box 8viii.1. Example of nutritional planning for 500 g neonatal puppy

Milk replacer nutritional density is 1 ml = 1 kcal:

(500g × 20– 26 kcal/day) /100 g = 120–130 kcal/day

Stomach capacity = 500 g × (1kg/ 1000 g) × (40– 50m l/1kg) = 20 – 25 ml

To avoid exceeding stomach capacity, feed 20 ml/meal.

Number of mealsper day = (120 kcal/day) / (20ml / meal) = 6 meals/day

2008). Patients who have low birth weights or who are hypothermic have higher needs and are also predisposed. The normal **blood sugar** in a neonate is reported to be 52–127 mg/dl for the first week of life (Munnich and Kuchenmeister, 2014). Hypoglycemia is prevalent in all pediatric patients (not just neonates), due to increased metabolic demand, limited glycogen storages, inefficient gluconeogenesis, poor response to glucagon, and reduced fat resulting in the inability to produce ketone bodies for fuel (Macintire, 2008; Lee and Cohn, 2017). Clinical signs associated with hypoglycemia include weakness, tremors, seizures, stupor, and coma.

Hypoglycemic crisis should be treated aggressively with intravenous or intraosseous 50% dextrose at 0.5–1 g/kg, diluted to a 5% solution (Macintire, 2008). Alternatively, 50% dextrose can be diluted with 1:3 sterile water to make a 12.5% dextrose solution and should be administered through a central line (to avoid phlebitis). Constant rate infusions of 2.5–5% dextrose in crystalloids can be used to maintain patients prone to or documented with hypoglycemia, given through a peripheral intravenous or intraosseous catheter. Over-supplementation with dextrose should be avoided, as it can lead to an osmotic diarrhea and subsequent worsening of dehydration (McMichael and Dhupa, 2000b; Lee and Cohn, 2017).

Supplementation with KCl at 20–30 mEq/l is often concurrently administered in the critically ill neonate (Lee and Cohn, 2017). See Chapters 7i and 7ii for additional information and practice calculations for dextrose and potassium supplementation.

8viii.10 Conclusion

The pediatric patient requires higher maintenance fluid therapy, due to their larger total body water content and propensity to develop hypovolemia and dehydration. While the oral route is preferred, aggressive intervention with intravenous or intraosseous catheterization can be life-saving in the severely affected patient. The veterinarian should consider goals of care, severity of disease, and patient age in order to tailor an individual fluid plan to the patient at hand.

References

Crawford, M.A. (1995) The urinary system. In: Hoskins, J.D. (ed.) *Veterinary Pediatrics: Dog and Cats from Birth to Six Months*, 2nd edn. W.B. Saunders, Philadelphia, Pennsylvania, pp. 271–292.

Faulks, R.D. and Lane, I.F. (2003) Qualitative urinalyses in puppies 0 to 24 weeks of age. *Journal of the American Animal Hospital Association* 39(4), 369–378.

Fettman, M.J. and Allen, T.A. (1991) Developmental aspects of fluid and electrolyte metabolism and renal function in neonates. *Compendium on Continuing Education for the Practicing Veterinarian (USA)* 13(3), 392.

Gunn-Moore, D. (2006) Techniques for neonatal resuscitation and critical care. In: *World Small Animal Veterinary Association World Congress Proceedings* (Prague), pp. 707–713.

Hoskins, J.D. (1995) Fluid therapy in the puppy and kitten. In: Kirk, R.W. (ed.) *Current Veterinary Therapy XII*, Vol. 1, 12th edn. W.B. Saunders, Philadelphia, Pennsylvania, pp. 34–37.

Jose, P.A., Slotkoff, L.M., Montgomery, S. *et al.* (1975) Autoregulation of renal blood flow in the puppy. *American Journal of Physiology–Legacy Content* 229(4), 983–988.

Kleinman, L.I. and Lubbe, R.J. (1972) Factors affecting the maturation of glomerular filtration rate and renal plasma flow in the new-born dog. *The Journal of Physiology* 223(2), 395–409.

Kleinman, L.I. and Reuter, J.H. (1974) Renal response of the new-born dog to a saline load: the role of intrarenal blood flow distribution. *The Journal of Physiology* 239(2), 225.

Laroute, V., Chetboul, V., Roche, L. *et al.* (2005) Quantitative evaluation of renal function in healthy Beagle puppies and mature dogs. *Research in Veterinary Science* 79(2), 161–167.

Lawler, D.F. (2008) Neonatal and pediatric care of the puppy and kitten. *Theriogenology* 70(3), 384–392.

Lee, J.A. and Cohn, L.A. (2017) Fluid therapy for pediatric patients. *Veterinary Clinics: Small Animal Practice* 47(2), 373–382.

Mace, S.E. and Levy, M.N. (1983) Neural control of heart rate: a comparison between puppies and adult animals. *Pediatric Research* 17(6), 491–495.

Macintire, D.K. (2008) Pediatric fluid therapy. *Veterinary Clinics of North America: Small Animal Practice* 38(3), 621–627.

McMichael, M. (2005) Pediatric emergencies. *Veterinary Clinics: Small Animal Practice* 35(2), 421–434.

McMichael, M. and Dhupa, N. (2000a) Pediatric critical care medicine: physiologic considerations. *Compendium on Continuing Education for the Practicing Veterinarian* 22(3), 206–214.

McMichael, M. and Dhupa, N. (2000b) Pediatric critical care medicine: specific syndromes. *Compendium on Continuing Education for the Practicing Veterinarian* 22(4), 353–359.

Munnich, A. and Kuchenmeister, U. (2014) Causes, diagnosis, and therapy of common diseases in neonatal puppies in the first days of life: cornerstones of practical approach. *Reproduction in Domestic Animals* 49, 64–74.

Poffenberger, E.M, Ralston, A.L., Chandler, M.L. *et al.* (1990) Canine neonatology: part 1. Physiologic differences between puppies and adults. *Compendium on Continuing Education for the Practicing Veterinarian* 12, 601–609.

8ix Special Considerations in Cats

Anda Young

The Ohio State University, Columbus, Ohio, USA

Feline patients requiring fluid therapy are common and the goal of euhydration should be approached with a few considerations in mind. Co-morbidities such as obesity, chronic kidney disease, and occult heart disease may predispose a feline patient to reduced tolerance of traditional methods of resuscitation, replacement, and maintenance fluid therapy (see Chapter 6). Additionally, select diseases such as urethral obstruction may lead to a phenomenon of post-obstructive diuresis which requires special considerations. With these idiosyncrasies in mind, fluid therapy in cats is approached utilizing tools such as low and slow resuscitation, hypotonic solutions for maintenance therapy, and early de-escalation strategies.

8ix.1 Obesity

Maintenance fluid requirements may be defined as the volume of fluid needed to achieve zero net gain of fluid accounting for measurable or sensible losses (e.g., urine) and immeasurable or insensible losses (respiratory, feces, saliva) (see Chapter 6iii for additional information). This fluid requirement has been estimated in certain settings based on daily energy (kcal) requirements, such that 1 ml of water is required for each kcal ingested. This estimation is based on observation of healthy research dogs where it was documented that water intake was found to be approximately 1 ml/kcal ingested. The physiologic basis for this association is hypothesized to be related to urinary losses associated with excretion of dietary solutes. Formulas used to derive the resting energy requirement and thus maintenance fluid requirement vary depending on the resource referenced. Given that caloric needs are a logarithmic function of body weight, it is of note that larger animals require less fluid than smaller animals. At the author's institution, the following formula is used to calculate resting energy requirement, which is extrapolated to provide daily maintenance water requirement (l/day) in feline patients (DiBartola, 2012):

Resting energy requirement (kcal/day) = body weight$_{(kg)}{}^{0.75}$ × 70–80

A limitation to using this approach is the fact that diets vary in dry matter content and energy composition (i.e., high-protein diets increase renal solute load more significantly than fat). Additionally, inconsistencies in consumption may be seen in the sick hyporexic patient. Further obstacles are met with the obese patient, as body composition is a major determinant of resting energy requirement, with adipose tissue being less metabolically active. Several human studies have documented higher resting energy expenditure in obese human patients; however, as compared with a lean population, differences in resting energy expenditure often abate once only highly metabolically active tissue weight is considered (Carneiro *et al.*, 2016). Obesity has also been associated with increased diuretic use in human critical care settings, a finding that correlated to sodium retention in a small sub-cohort (de Louw *et al.*, 2015). Evidence is lacking to suggest that obese patients have increased fluid therapy requirements and, given potential to do harm, it is recommended to calculate maintenance fluid rates based on lean body weight to avoid attainment of a positive fluid balance.

Feline daily fluid requirement (ml/day)
= lean body weight$_{(kg)}{}^{0.75}$ × 70

Clinical Case 8ix.1 gives an example of fluid therapy in the obese patient.

8ix.2 Occult Heart Disease

Normal methods of screening for cardiac disease (e.g., cardiac auscultation, thoracic radiography) may not be reliable in feline patients, due to the nature of their commonly acquired cardiomyopathy, **hypertrophic cardiomyopathy** (HCM). The first limitation with such screening tools is that murmurs in the feline population may be dynamic (i.e., changing

DOI: 10.1079/9781789243406.0089

Clinical Case 8ix.1. Fluid therapy in the obese patient

A 7-year-old FS domestic medium-hair cat weighing 9 kg presents for anorexia of 3 days duration and hiding behavior. The patient is strictly indoor, eats a mixed dry kibble and wet food diet. The patient intermittently vomits hair balls; no other pertinent history is reported. On physical examination the patient is considered to be ≤5% dehydrated and obese with a 9/9 body condition score (ideal 5/9). Heart sounds are difficult to auscult clearly, due to patient size; no gallop or heart murmur is detected. There is general malaise and pyrexia (103.1°F/39.5°C), but the remainder of the examination is considered unremarkable. The following diagnostics are obtained at the time of presentation.

Parameter	Value	S.I. (US)	Reference low	Reference high
Plasma protein	75 (7.50)	g/l (g/dl)	56 (5.6)	83 (8.3)
HCT	43	%	27	45
Hemoglobin	143 (14.3)	g/l (g/dl)	92 (9.2)	153 (15.3)
RBC	10.13 (10.13)	× 10^9/l (×10^3/μl)	6.3 (6.3)	10.6 (10.6)
MCV	43 (43)	fl (μm^3)	38 (38)	48 (48)
MCHC	331 (33.1)	g/l (g/dl)	332 (33.2)	361 (36.1)
RDW	14.40	%	13.7	17.5
Reticulocyte – absolute	90.1 (90.1)	× 10^9/l (×10^3/μl)	0	105
Platelet count	156 (156)	× 10^9/l (×10^3/μl)	128 (128)	444 (444)
MPV	18.6 (18.6)	fl (μm^3)	9.8 (9.8)	21.9 (21.9)
Total leukocytes	20.2 (20.2) *	× 10^9/l (×10^3/μl)	2.3 (2.3)	18.4 (18.4)
Segmented neutrophils	12.6 (12.6) *	× 10^9/l (×10^3/μl)	1.4 (1.4)	11.8 (11.8)
Lymphocytes	4.9 (4.9)	× 10^9/l (×10^3/μl)	0.6 (0.6)	5.7 (5.7)
Monocytes	0.20 (0.20)	× 10^9/l (×10^3/μl)	0 (0)	0.6 (0.6)
Eosinophils	1.21 (1.21)	× 10^9/l (×10^3/μl)	0 (0)	1.5 (1.5)
BUN	10.7 (30.0) *	mmol/l (mg/dl)	3.57 (10)	9.64 (27)
Creatinine	122 (1.60) *	μmol/l (mg/dl)	7.63 (0.1)	99.1 (1.3)
Phosphorus	1.1 (3.4)	mmol/l (mg/dl)	0.71 (2.2)	2.03 (6.3)
Calcium – total	2.38 (9.5)	mmol/l (mg/dl)	2.27 (9.1)	2.88 (11.5)
Sodium	145 (145)	mmol/l (mEq/l)	145 (145)	154 (154)
Potassium	3.9 (3.9)	mmol/l (mEq/l)	3.9 (3.9)	5.5 (5.5)
Chloride	111 (111)	mmol/l (mEq/l)	107 (107)	118 (118)
Anion Gap	20 (20)	mmol/l (mEq/l)	15 (15)	25 (25)
Osmolality (calc)	325 (325) *	mmol/kg (mOsm/kg)	289 (289)	308 (308)
Bicarbonate – total	18.1 (18.1)	mmol/l (mEq/l)	18 (18)	27 (27)
ALT – alanine amino transferase	3.84 (230) *	μkat/l (IU/l)	0.3 (18)	1.8 (108)
AST – aspartate amino transferase	2.14 (128) *	μkat/l (IU/l)	0.27 (16)	0.85 (51)
AP – alkaline phosphatase	7.51 (450) *	μkat/l (IU/l)	0.2 (12)	2.22 (133)
CK – creatine kinase	1.49 (89)	μkat/l (IU/l)	0.89 (53)	6.21 (372)
Cholesterol	11.4 (440) *	mmol/l (mg/dl)	3.16 (122)	8.94 (345)
Bilirubin – total	8.55 (0.5) *	μmol/l (mg/dl)	0.86 (0.05)	3.42 (0.2)
Total protein – Serum	80 (8.0) *	g/l (g/dl)	51 (5.1)	71 (7.1)
Albumin	40 (4.0)	g/l (g/dl)	3.3 (0.33)	4.2 (0.42)
Globulin	32 (3.2)	G'l (g/dl)	17 (1.7)	34 (3.4)
Glucose – Serum	13 (234)*	mmol/l (mg/dl)	3.72 (67)	7.05 (127)
GGT	0.17 (10)	μkat/l (IU/l)	0 (0)	0.37 (22.3)

* Abnormal value, outside the reference range.

Continued

Clinical Case 8ix.1. Continued.

The patient is diagnosed with an acute liver injury with a primary differential of cholangiohepatitis and is hospitalized in ICU for overnight hydration prior to the acquisition of an abdominal ultrasound and liver aspirates. Given the obese nature of the patient, the following calculations are used to generate a fluid therapy plan.

1. Body condition calculations:
   (Patient body condition) – (Ideal body condition)
   9 – 5 = 4
   Excess body weight calculation: 10% for each excess body condition point
   10% × 4 = 40%
   Lean body weight calculation
   9 kg × 0.60 = 5.6 kg lean body weight
2. Rehydration fluid rate:
   0.05 × 5.6 kg = 280 ml deficit correct over 36 h = 7 ml/h
3. Maintenance fluid rate:
   $\mathbf{5.6^{0.75}}$ × 70 = 254 ml/day ÷ 24 h/day = 10 ml/h
4. Total fluid rate:
   10 ml/h + 7 ml/h = 17 ml/h

in intensity) or intermittent. Additionally, there is diversity in the etiology of a murmur, including structural heart disease, high cardiac output (i.e., anemia, hyperthyroidism, high sympathetic tone) or non-pathologic "innocent" murmurs. In general populations, it has been documented that approximately one-third of cats will have murmurs (Wagner *et al*., 2010). Of those with murmurs, approximately 30–60% will have echocardiographic measurements of left ventricular hypertrophy (Wagner *et al*., 2010). In referral populations, 53% of apparently healthy cats presenting to a cardiology service for evaluation of a heart murmur had echocardiographic evidence of cardiac disease (Nakamura *et al*., 2011). It is of note that as a cat progresses from a juvenile to senior life stage, the prevalence of a murmur representing structural heart disease increases from approximately 18% to 43% (Luis Fuentes and Wilkie, 2017). On the contrary, lack of a murmur does not eliminate the possibility of structural heart disease, as 7–28% of cats screened and diagnosed with hypertrophic cardiomyopathy did not have a murmur (Luis Fuentes and Wilkie, 2017). Physical examination findings such as an audible gallop sound are more specific for HCM, given the representation of diastolic dysfunction. Additionally, an arrhythmia may suggest underlying structural heart disease, as its presence has been linked to cardiac-related mortality (Luis Fuentes and Wilkie, 2017).

Cardiac biomarkers such as N-terminal pro-brain natriuretic peptide (NT-proBNP) offer insight into at-risk populations. BNP is secreted from atrial and ventricular myocytes during myocardial stretch or neurohormonal stimuli. NT-proBNP is constitutively produced by the myocardium and its release has been shown to correlate with measures of disease severity (i.e., left ventricular wall thickness, left atrial size). The point-of-care (POC) NT-proBNP ELISA tests prove most reliable in diagnosing moderate to severe cardiomyopathy in higher-risk populations. False negatives, albeit uncommon, are possible in cats with moderate disease. False-positive results are possible in cats with mild cardiomyopathy, or co-morbidities such as chronic kidney disease (CKD) or non-cardiac respiratory disease (Loughran *et al*., 2019). As such, positive point-of-care testing warrants definitive testing with echocardiogram (Machen *et al*., 2014). In the absence of gold-standard echocardiography, focused cardiac ultrasound performed by non-specialist practitioners has been shown to be useful for increasing the level of suspicion that a feline patient has moderate to severe cardiomyopathy (Loughran *et al*., 2019). Interestingly, this same study showed that a focused ultrasound was non-inferior to focused ultrasound plus point-of-care BNP testing in diagnosing occult heart disease. Such bedside testing may continue to serve the emergency clinician by increasing their level of concern for occult cardiomyopathy patients.

When parenteral fluid therapy is indicated in the cardiac patient or suspected cardiac patient, solutions that are hypotonic to the patient (i.e., 0.45% NaCl or D5W) should be considered for provision of maintenance fluid requirement, as excessive sodium load can increase the risk of overload. In this context 0.45% NaCl can be thought of as approximately 50% free water as compared with the patient. Dextrose 5% in water contains no sodium, thus contains 100% free water as compared to the patient. Free water will distribute into all fluid compartments: intravascular, interstitial, and intracellular spaces. As such, use of hypotonic fluids opens the intracellular compartment for fluid entry, offloading the intravascular, interstitial, and thus cardiovascular system. Isotonic crystalloids, on the other hand, contain salt and water in equal parts as compared with the patient. These fluids will only distribute across the extracellular space, thereby potentially increasing the risk for the development of interstitial edema in states of cardiac insufficiency. However, these fluids can be used to cautiously replace isotonic losses.

With the use of hypotonic fluids, sodium and potassium levels should be monitored periodically. If hyponatremia or hypokalemia develop, crystalloid solution and electrolyte supplementation should be adjusted accordingly. Additionally, patients at risk for congestive heart failure or fluid overload should be monitored hourly for changes in respiratory rates and effort. Serial assessment of body weight every 6–8 h can also assist in providing objective parameters that rehydration goals have been achieved.

Clinical Case 8ix.2 gives an example of suspect cardiomyopathy.

8ix.3 Urethral Obstruction

Feline urethral obstruction continues to be a frequent presenting complaint that requires emergency intervention and hospitalization. Risk factors for urethral obstruction (UO) including male sex, older age, increased body condition, indoor lifestyle, and eating a predominantly dry diet have been reported (Gerber *et al.*, 2008; Jukes *et al.*, 2019). The etiology of UO has changed over the years. It has been accepted over the past decade that the most common cause of UO is feline interstitial cystitis followed by urolithiasis and urethral plug, with a minority of cases being caused by stricture or neoplasia (Gerber *et al.*, 2008). The survival to discharge remains high (90–95%), but in-hospital morbidity associated with electrolyte derangements, post-obstructive diuresis or volume overload has been reported (Francis *et al.*, 2010; Cooper, 2015; Frohlich *et al.*, 2016;Ostroski *et al.*, 2017).

Severe electrolyte derangements are not uncommon in patients experiencing complete UO as a result of reduced glomerular filtration and urine retention. This leads to accumulation of blood urea nitrogen, creatinine, phosphorus, potassium, and hydrogen ions. The resulting uremic toxicosis leads to the clinical signs observed by the owner and clinician, including nausea, anorexia, vomiting, and depression (Drobatz *et al.*, 2019). In patients in which treatment is delayed, severe hyperkalemia can lead to fatal arrhythmias secondary to disturbed

Clinical Case 8ix.2. Cardiomyopathy suspect

A 14-year-old FS domestic shorthair with a chronic history of inflammatory bowel disease presents for a 4-day history of progressive diarrhea. On physical examination the patient weighs 4.9 kg with a 3/9 body condition score and is determined to be approximately 7% dehydrated. A grade IV/VI left parasternal systolic heart murmur is detected. The following diagnostics are obtained at the time of presentation:

Parameter	Value	S.I. (US)	Reference low	Reference high
PCV	43	%	27	45
Total protein	86 (8.6)	g/l (g/dl)	56 (5.6)	83 (8.3)

The patient is hospitalized in ICU for rehydration and supportive care therapy. Given the high risk for undiagnosed cardiomyopathy in this patient, the following calculations were used to generate a fluid therapy plan:

1. Replacement of dehydration (isotonic losses):
   4.9 kg x 0.07 = 0.343 l deficit over 36 h = 10 ml/h administered with balanced crystalloid
2. Maintenance fluid rate:
   $\mathbf{4.9^{0.75}}$ x 70 = 230 ml/day ÷ 24 h/day = 9 ml/h administered with 0.45% NaCl
3. Total fluid rate:
   9.5 ml/h balanced crystalloid + 9 ml/h 0.45% NaCl = 19 ml/h

Given the concern for underlying cardiac disease, a longer time-frame for replacement of dehydration is selected (36 h). Also, given the subjectivity in hydration assessment in older felines with reduced fat stores, careful monitoring is instituted with serial body weight measurement. The patient is estimated to have a 0.343 l deficit, which equates to 0.343 kg. The patient will be weighed every 6–8 h with call parameters to alert the clinician once the patient has gained 7% of baseline body weight (5.2 kg), at which time the patient should be re-evaluated for hydration assessment and fluid therapy modification. Serial monitoring of PCV/TP may also be of benefit.

Clinical Case 8ix.3. Post-obstructive diuresis

A 5-year-old strictly indoor neutered male domestic shorthair cat weighing 5.5 kg presents with a history of straining in the litterbox and progressive lethargy over 24 h. The patient is examined to be approximately 6% dehydrated with a heart rate of 140 and a painful, firm distended bladder. The patient is diagnosed with circulatory shock and a urethral obstruction. Laboratory work reveals hyperkalemia and associated electrocardiogram changes are addressed with calcium gluconate and a conservative fluid bolus followed by replacement fluid therapy (see Chapter 7iii for a case scenario of hyperkalemia secondary to feline urethral obstruction). A moderate post-renal azotemia is detected. No historical renal values are available for the patient.

Following stabilization, the patient is successfully de-obstructed, and the urinary bladder is emptied to allow for a zero net baseline. The patient is monitored with telemetry for 6–8 h as replacement + maintenance fluid therapy is administered, and urine output is collected in a closed collection system. Cardiac re-evaluation is performed; no heart murmur or gallop rhythm is detected. The patient is considered to have a good body condition thus fluid rate calculations are performed using the measured body weight of 5.5 kg. A rehydration correction rate is arbitrarily chosen, taking into account the rate at which volume losses occurred and the patient's tolerance of generous fluid rates (i.e., no occult cardiomyopathy, underlying CKD or concern for acute on chronic kidney injury, etc.)

1. Rehydration fluid rate:
   5.5 kg × 0.06 = 0.330 l deficit over 18 h = 18 ml/h
2. Maintenance fluid rate:
   $5.5\ kg^{0.75} \times 70 = 10$ ml/h
3. Total fluid rate:
   18 ml/h + 10 ml/h = 28 ml/h

Four hours following the unblocking procedure, the patient's urine output is quantified to observe for low urine production (<1–2 ml/kg/h) or the development of a post-obstructive diuresis (urinary output in excess of expected fluid therapy induced diuresis).

Low urine production could suggest a few things, as follows.

a) Equipment malfunction. The urinary catheter could be obstructed with blood clots, cellular debris or grit/crystals/calculi. Instilling sterile flush in a retrograde fashion can dislodge such debris. The urinary catheter can also become wedged against the urinary bladder as the bladder shrinks down around the tip. The catheter may need to be backed out so that it terminates in the urinary bladder trigone. Urine flow should resume once it is backed out to an appropriate location.

b) Low effective circulating volume. If the patient continues to have low effective circulating volume from severe dehydration this may manifest as low urinary output. The urinary specific gravity is specific (USG >1.050 reflects dehydration) but poorly sensitive, such that a lower USG could be the result of the disturbed intramedullary concentrating gradients that occur during urethral obstruction. In this scenario the clinician has the option to stay the course with the rehydration plan or increase the rate at which dehydration is corrected.

c) Intrinsic renal injury-related oliguria/anuria. If a patient has pre-existing kidney disease and subsequently experiences a post-renal acute kidney injury, low urine output could represent intrinsic oliguria/anuria in which there are insufficient functional nephrons available to form ultrafiltrate and thus produce urine. This remains a diagnosis of exclusion once options (a) and (b) have been addressed.

The patient's urine output 4 h following obstruction relief is 209 ml, which equates to 52 ml/h or 9.5 ml/kg/h. Because these urinary losses exceed the amount of fluid given and are far more than would be expected in a dehydrated patient early in the course of fluid therapy, this patient is exhibiting signs of a post-obstructive diuresis. Unmatched it could lead to further dehydration and hypovolemia. At this point in time the patient is weighed and is assessed for cardiovascular stability. If he has lost weight since admission or is determined to be severely dehydrated or exhibiting signs of hypovolemic shock, a conservative fluid bolus (e.g., balanced crystalloid at 5 ml/kg over 30 min) could be administered. However, he is deemed to be stable, and so the decision is made to start adjusting the fluid rate to match urinary output:

1. Quantify OUTs
   209 ml/h ÷ 4 h = 52 ml/h
2. Match fluid rate to urinary output
   New fluid rate = 52 ml/h. As mentioned above, while typically ongoing losses would be added to maintenance, this would *not* be done here.
3. Repeat steps (1) and (2) in 4 h.

Matching INs and OUTs are continued and within 18 h the patient is determined to be euhydrated and laboratory values (BUN, creatinine, potassium) have normalized. The patient is still producing urine at approximately 40 ml/h (7.2 ml/kg/h). It is then decided to taper fluids based on urine production, returning only 80%:

Urine output = 40 ml/h × 0.8 = 32 ml/h

This adjustment is made every 4 h and over the next 12 h the urine output decreases and reaches a rate of 15 ml/h (2.7 ml/kg/h). At this time the decision is made to remove his urinary catheter and his fluid rate is decreased to maintenance (10 ml/h).

cardiac electrophysiology (see Chapter 7ii). This manifests as prolonged PR interval or blunted to absent P waves, widened QRS complexes, and tall tented T waves (Parham *et al.*, 2006). It should be noted that electrocardiogram changes are poorly sensitive for alterations in serum potassium levels and normal or subtly altered tracings can be seen in feline patients with potassium levels that exceed 8.5 mEq/l (Tag and Day, 2008). However, ECG tracings can help dictate which hyperkalemia interventions are selected with urgency.

Albeit counter-intuitive in a patient that is unable to urinate, intravenous fluid therapy is considered first-line therapy in stabilizing felines with UO, as it serves to dilute serum [K], support effective circulating volume, and address metabolic derangement. Urethral obstruction patients presenting in shock are often suffering from reduced effective circulating volume (ECV), as they are often fluid responsive. The reduced ECV is likely multi-factorial, including reduced water intake and volume loss through the GI tract secondary to vomiting, respectively. Additionally, bradyrhythms and altered vascular tone may result from hyperkalemia and metabolic derangements (i.e., hypocalcemia, metabolic acidosis). In human medicine, bladder distention can independently lead to autonomic vaso-vagal reflexes manifesting as vomiting, bradycardia, hypotension, hypertension, cardiac dysrhythmias, or even asystole (Prakash *et al.*, 2014; Al-Sadawi *et al.*, 2019). Any crystalloid available to the clinician is appropriate for stabilization and initial patient management. Alkalinizing balanced crystalloids (e.g., Plasma-Lyte, lactated Ringer's) are non-inferior to 0.9% NaCl in treating hyperkalemia and may lead to more rapid resolution of acid–base derangements (Drobatz and Cole, 2008; Cunha *et al.*, 2010). Despite faster resolution of acid–base disturbances, patient outcomes are reported to be similar regardless of crystalloid choice, emphasizing the point that any crystalloid is considered appropriate for patient stabilization. Volume resuscitation is administered through bolus doses (i.e., 5–10 ml/kg) administered over 15–30 min (see Chapter 6i). At the author's institution, once the patient is determined to be euvolemic, the hydration status is estimated, and initial fluid rates are established based on correction of dehydration + maintenance. It is prudent to re-assess the patient in 4–6 h for urine output and tolerance of fluid therapy, as those who develop a post-obstructive diuresis may require frequent adjustment of fluid rates.

Post-obstructive diuresis (POD) is characterized as increased urine production (> 2 ml/kg/h) following resolution of a urinary obstruction. The pathogenesis is not completely understood, but it may be related to retention of uremic osmoles, tubular injury and dysfunction, medullary washout, antidiuretic hormone resistance, and increases in natriuretic hormones (Cooper, 2015). In experimental rat studies of bilateral ureteral ligation, POD typically develops within 2–3 h of obstruction resolution, lasting up to 30 days (Frohlich *et al.*, 2016). Retrospective feline UO studies looking at predictors of conventionally defined POD are difficult to interpret, given concurrent fluid therapy-induced diuresis. One study attempted to define a POD more objectively as two consecutive net loss urine output measurements. When this definition was used, the incidence of POD developing within the first 12 h approximated 30%. Two studies have found significant correlation between acidemia and the development of a POD, while no correlation has been found with regard to BUN, creatinine or electrolytes (Francis *et al.*, 2010; Frohlich *et al.*, 2016). Rates of urine production can be significant in the face of POD and could lead to significant dehydration and hypovolemia if left unchecked. In this regard, frequent quantification of urine output (every 4–8 h) is important to help adjust fluid rate accordingly. Matching the hourly urine output can help to ensure that urinary losses are met. It is important to note that a maintenance fluid rate should not be added to these urinary losses. As normal urinary losses constitute the majority of maintenance fluid needs, this would essentially be giving that portion twice. The result would be a progressive escalation of urine output/fluid rate and should be avoided. See Clinical Case 8ix.3 for additional explanation.

Post-obstructive diuresis generates high tubular flow rates and can therefore lead to substantial reductions in serum potassium levels. As such, renal and electrolyte values should be monitored at least every 12 h during the first 24–48 h and supplemented accordingly. Once these parameters have normalized, fluid therapy can be tapered by matching only some portion of the urine produced (e.g. 75–80%). The urine output should slowly taper in response to gentle fluid reductions until more normal urine outputs of 2–4 ml/kg/h are achieved. In the author's experience, a true post-obstructive diuresis resolves over the course of a few days but may certainly take longer in certain scenarios.

References

Al-Sadawi, M., Garcia, A.N., Ihsan, M. *et al.* (2019) Bladder distension: an overlooked cause vagal-induced hypotension during coronary angiography. *American Journal of Medical Case Reports* 7, 180–183.

Carneiro, I.P., Elliott, S.A., Siervo, M. *et al.* (2016) Is obesity associated with altered energy expenditure? *Advanced Nutrition* 7, 476–487.

Cooper, E.S. (2015) Controversies in the management of feline urethral obstruction. *Journal of Veterinary Emergency and Critical Care* 25, 130–137.

Cunha, M.G., Freitas, G.C., Carregaro, A.B. *et al.* (2010) Renal and cardiorespiratory effects of treatment with lactated Ringer's solution or physiologic saline (0.9% NaCl) solution in cats with experimentally induced urethral obstruction. *American Journal of Veterinary Research* 71, 840–846.

de Louw, E.J., Sun, P.O., Lee, J. *et al.* (2015) Increased incidence of diuretic use in critically ill obese patients. *Journal of Critical Care* 30, 619–623.

DiBartola, S.P. (ed.) (2012) *Fluid, Electrolyte, and Acid–Base Disorders in Small Animal Practice*, 4th edn. Saunders/Elsevier, St Louis, Missouri.

Drobatz, K.J. and Cole, S.G. (2008) The influence of crystalloid type on acid–base and electrolyte status of cats with urethral obstruction. *Journal of Veterinary Emergency and Critical Care* 18, 355–361.

Drobatz, K.J., Hopper, K., Rozanski, E.A. and Silverstein, D.C. (eds) (2019) *Textbook of Small Animal Emergency Medicine*. John Wiley and Sons, Hoboken, New Jersey.

Francis, B.J., Wells, R.J., Rao, S. and Hackett, TB. (2010) Retrospective study to characterize post-obstructive diuresis in cats with urethral obstruction. *Journal of Feline Medicine and Surgery* 12, 606–608.

Frohlich, L., Hartmann, K., Sautter-Loius, C. and Dorsch, R. (2016) Postobstructive diuresis in cats with naturally occurring lower urinary tract obstruction: incidence, severity and association with laboratory parameters on admission. *Journal of Feline Medicine and Surgery* 18, 809–817.

Gerber, B., Eichenberger, S. and Reusch, C.E. (2008) Guarded long-term prognosis in male cats with urethral obstruction. *Journal of Feline Medicine and Surgery* 10, 16–23.

Jukes, A., Lui, M., Morton, J.M. *et al.* (2019) Associations between increased body condition score, bodyweight, age and breed with urethral obstruction in male castrated cats. *Veterinary Journal* 244, 7–12.

Loughran, K.A., Rush, J.E., Rozanski, E.A. *et al.* (2019) The use of focused cardiac ultrasound to screen for occult heart disease in asymptomatic cats. *Journal of Veterinary Internal Medicine* 33, 1892–1901.

Luis Fuentes, V. and Wilkie, L.J. (2017) Asymptomatic hypertrophic cardiomyopathy: diagnosis and therapy. *Veterinary Clinics of North America Small Animal Practice* 47, 1041–1054.

Machen, M.C., Oyama, M.A., Gordon, S.G. *et al.* (2014) Multi-centered investigation of a point-of-care NT-proBNP ELISA assay to detect moderate to severe occult (pre-clinical) feline heart disease in cats referred for cardiac evaluation. *Journal of Veterinary Cardiology* 16, 245–255.

Nakamura, R.K., Rishniw, M., King, M.K. *et al.* (2011) Prevalence of echocardiographic evidence of cardiac disease in apparently healthy cats with murmurs. *Journal of Feline Medicine and Surgery* 13, 266–271.

Ostroski, C.J., Drobatz, K.J. and Reineke, E.L. (2017) Retrospective evaluation of and risk factor analysis for presumed fluid overload in cats with urethral obstruction: 11 cases (2002–2012). *Journal of Veterinary Emergency and Critical Care* 27, 561–568.

Parham, W.A., Mehdirad, A.A., Biermann, K.M. and Fredman, C.S. (2006) Hyperkalemia revisited. *Texas Heart Institute Journal* 33, 40–47.

Prakash, S., Kael, S., Mullick, P. and Gogia, A.R. (2014) Cardiovascular manifestations of perioperative acute urinary bladder over-distension. *Indian Journal of Anaesthesiology* 58, 502–504.

Tag, T.L. and Day, T.K. (2008) Electrocardiographic assessment of hyperkalemia in dogs and cats. *Journal of Veterinary Emergency and Critical Care* 18, 61–67.

Wagner, T., Fuentes, V.L., Payne, J.R. *et al.* (2010) Comparison of auscultatory and echocardiographic findings in healthy adult cats. *Journal of Veterinary Cardiology* 12, 171–182.

Index

Note: The page numbers in *italics* and **bold** represents figures and tables respectively.

activated clotting time (ACT) *29*
acute hyponatremia 119
acute kidney injury (AKI) 18
  clinical case 112–114
  clinical approach 111
  GFR 110
  maintenance phase 112
  overzealous fluid administration 110
  polyuria 110
  positive fluid balance 111
  removal phase 112
  resuscitation 111–112
  urine parameters 110
acute traumatic coagulopathy (ATC) 96
ADH *see* antidiuretic hormone
AKI *see* acute kidney injury
albumin 27
  blood products, in veterinary medicine **28**
  canine plasma product 31
  clinical effects, intravenous solutions **28**
  coagulopathy, ACT *29*
  cryo-poor plasma 28
  definition 27
  FFP 29
  HSA use 30
  hypoalbuminemia 27, 30
  transfusion reaction to plasma 29–30
  veterinary sources 28
amylopectin 19
anemic shock 42, 46
anesthesia/perioperative
  analgesic and anesthetic drugs 117
  balanced isotonic crystalloids 115
  clinical cases 117–118
  crystalloid bolus 117
  crystalloid/colloid/blood product 117
  dynamic indices 117
  fluid administration 115
  fluid bolus 117
  hypotension during anesthesia *116*
  hypotensive patient **116**
  monitoring fluid resuscitation 117
  perioperative fluid administration 115
angiotensin II 56
antidiuretic hormone (ADH) 119, 126

beta-2 adrenergic agonist 76
blood urea nitrogen (BUN) 57
body fluid compartments
  electrolytes, between ICS/ECS *4*
  extracellular fluid balance, risk of edema formation **8**
  extracellular space 3
  glycocalyx 7, *8*
  intracellular/extracellular compartments, movement between 3–4
  intravascular/interstitial compartments, movement between 5–7
  osmotic gradients, movement of water *5*
  starling equation 6, *6*
  starling forces, values **6**
  total body water 3
  water distribution *4*

calcium/phosphorus homeostasis
  causes 83
  clinical cases
    clinical cases 86–87
    hyperkalemia 85–86
    periparturient hypocalcemia 87–88
    phosphorus supplementation, diabetic ketoacidosis 88–90
  hormonal influences *82*
  hormonal regulation, Ca
    biological roles 81
    parathyroid glands 81
    PTH 81
  hormonal regulation, Pi 82
  hypercalcemia, severity in dogs/cats *83*
  hyperphosphatemia/hypophosphatemia causes **84**
  hypocalcemia, severity in dogs/cats *84*
  parenteral calcium solutions/dosing information **85**
  PTH effector organs 82–83
  supplementation 83–85
cardiac biomarkers 135
cardiac/kidney disease 39
catecholamines 68
cats, fluid therapy
  cardiomyopathy, clinical case 136–137
  feline urethral obstruction 136, 138
  maintenance fluid requirements 133

cats, fluid therapy (*continued*)
obese patients, clinical case 134–135
obesity 133
occult heart disease
BNP testing 135
cardiac disease 133
gold-standard echocardiography 135
hyponatremia/hypokalemia 136
isotonic crystalloids 136
parenteral fluid therapy 135
central nervous system 68
central/peripheral venous catheter 33–35
central pontine demyelination (CPD) 119
chronic kidney disease (CKD) 40, 111, 135
"classic" approach 98
colloid osmotic pressure (COP) 20, 26, 123
colloids 128
natural 26–31
synthetic 18–24
constant vs continuous rate infusion (CRI) 28, 70, 78, 83, 94, 104, 124, 131
COP *see* colloid osmotic pressure
"COP paradox" 21
cryo-poor plasma (CPP) 26, 103, 124
crystalloids
acid–base balance 10
hypertonic (*see* hypertonic crystalloids)
hypotonic (*see* hypotonic crystalloids)
isotonic (*see* isotonic crystalloids)

dehydration
clinical assessment 54
decision-making process, rehydrate patients
administration route 58, *59*
fluid selection 57
monitoring endpoints 59
rate of administration 58–59
excessive insensible water losses 54
extracellular fluid compartment, loss *57*
isotonic crystalloid fluids **58**
laboratory findings 56–57
physical examination 54, **55**
body weight, changes 55–56
hydration parameter 55
hypovolemia signs 56
mucous membrane moistness 55
position of eye, orbit 55, *56*
shock 55
skin elasticity 55
thirst 56
replace ongoing losses 59–60
respiratory losses 54
systemic approach 61
dextrans 18, 22
dextrose supplementation
buretrol, smaller volume *70*
diagnostic evaluation 68–69
glucose utilization/regulation 68
hypoglycemia, causes 68
monitoring/discontinuing supplementation 70–71
symptomatic patient, treatment 69–70

early goal-directed therapy (EGDT) 48
effective circulating volume (ECV) 138
electrocardiogram (ECG) 43
endothelial glycocalyx (EG) 2, 7, 8, 21, 49
endothelial surface layer (ESL) 3, 6, 8, 21
enteral route (EN) 33
GI tract 39
maintenance fluid requirement 39
extracellular fluid (ECF) 54, 73

fluid resuscitation
algorithm *50*
characteristics 47
classic approach 47–48
classic/revised doses **48**
clinical case 51–52
monitoring 49–51
pressure bags, intravenous fluids *47*
replacement phase, dehydration 54
revised approach 48–49
routes of administration 46–47
shock
anemic shock 42
causes **42**
clinical signs 43–44
diagnostics 44
hypoglycemia 42
hypovolemia 41
normal cardiovascular homeostasis 41
pathogenesis 41
perfusion parameters **43**
preload 41
types of fluid **45,** 45–46
fresh frozen plasma (FFP) 26, 103, 124
fresh whole blood (FWB) 26, *27*

gastrointestinal losses 54
gelatins 19
GFR *see* glomerular filtrate rate
glomerular filtrate rate (GFR) 110
glucagon 68
gravity-fed system 36

heart diseases
clinical cases 108–109
conjunctival edema, due to fluid overload *108*
counter-regulatory mechanisms 107

fluid overload, signs 108
fluid therapy administration 107
intravenous medications 107
serum electrolytes, serial monitoring 107
hemorrhage/trauma
acute hemorrhage, classification **96**
bleeding patients 98
blood products 101
"classic" approach 98
clinical cases 100–101
fluid resuscitation *99*
fluid types 96–98, **97**
"lethal triad" *96*
"massive transfusion" 98
monitoring/resuscitation endpoints 100
plasma proteins *95*
red blood cells *95*
trauma/bleeding patients, revised fluid does/rates **99**
traumatic injury *95*
HTS *see* hypertonic saline
human serum albumin (HSA) 30, 31, 104
hydroxyethyl starch (HES)
acute volume expansion 23, 24
albumin 21
C2 and C6 positions, substitution 20
concentration 20
definition 19
degree of substitution 20
human populations 23
hydroxyethyl substitution 20, *20*
hypoalbuminemia 23
indications/contraindications 23–24
MW 20
serum amylase activity 21
VetStarch *19*
hyperkalemia
cardiac effects 74
renal/adrenal function 74
RMP 74
treatment
cardioprotective effects 74
cardiovascular collapse 74
causes **75**
cystocentesis 76
emergency dosing **75**
hypernatremia
causes 120
clinical case 121–122
definition 120
hyperosmolality 120
loss of free water 120
rate for correction 120
treatment 120
hypertonic crystalloids 45
acute hyponatremia 15
adverse effects 16
applications *16*
composition **15**
concentration *15*
dehydration 16
hypertonic saline (HTS) 14, 97
sodium load, avoid patients 17
hypertrophic cardiomyopathy (HCM) 133
hypoalbuminemia 128
hypocalcemia 81
hypokalemia
cats, with severe hypokalemia *77*
causes **76**
clinical cases 79
definition 76
fatal effects 77
monitoring 79
potassium supplementation chart **78**
symptoms 76
treatment 77–78
hypokalemic polymyopathy 76, 77
hypomagnesia 91
hyponatremia
acute plasma 119
ADH 119
causes 120
chronic hyponatremia 119
chronic severe 119
clinical case 121
definition 119
"replace" sodium 119
sodium content 120
hypoproteinemia
clinical cases 124–125
colloids 123
concentrated canine albumin 124
dehydration 123
fluid therapy plan 123
formula- driven dosing 124
hypoalbuminemia 124
hypoalbuminemia patients 123
leakage of fluid 123
natural colloids 124
synthetic colloids 123, 124
synthetic molecules 123
hypoproteinemia/hypoalbuminemi 103
hypotension 43–44, 115
hypotonic crystalloids 45
composition **11**
contraindications/adverse effects 12
effective osmolarity 10
electrolytes 10
examples 10, *11*
free water deficit 10
total body water 10
use 10–12
hypotonic fluids 123
hypovolemia 103, 126, 127
hypoxemic shock 42

insulin 68
intracellular fluid (ICF) 73
intracellular fluid dehydration 54
intracranial pressure (ICP) 15
intraoperative fluid therapy 115
intraosseous route (IO) 33
catheter types 37
disadvantages 37, 38
drill system *37*
medullary cavity 37
placement of IO needle *37*
intraperitoneal fluid administration 129
intravenous catheter 30, 100
intravenous (IV) route 33
administer 33
administration 35–37
central venous 35
complications 37
distinct lumens, cross-sectional arrangement *35*
examples 35–37, *36*
peripheral catheters 34, *35*
triple-lumen central catheter *35*
types 33
ionized calcium (iCa) 81
isotonic crystalloids 45, 51, 111, 127, 136
acid–base balance 12, 14
adverse effects 14
balanced electrolyte solutions 13
buffering/alkalinizing effect 13
composition **12**
electrolyte composition 12
examples *13*
fluids 65, 115, 123
therapy 76
use 13–14

lactate-based or acetate/gluconate-based fluid 103
lactated Ringer's solution (LRS) 13, *57*, 58, 115
lyophilized canine albumin 103

magnesium
bone storage accounts 91
causes of hypomagnesemia **92**
clinical hypomagnesemia 92–94
clinical case 93
clinical signs 91–92
companion animals **92**
diagnosis 91
emergency treatment, intravenous magnesium *92*
GI tract 91
numerous cellular metabolic processes 91
magnesium sulfate (MgSO4) *92*
maintenance fluid therapy 11
bicarbonate precursors 66
clinical cases 66–67
commercial maintenance 66
crystalloids 65
dextrose 66
electrolyte status 65
hypotonic crystalloids 63
hypotonic crystalloids, compared with plasma **64**
hypotonic fluid *65*
isotonic fluids 67
phases 63
physiological losses 63
requirement 63–65, **64**
malabsorptive disorders 123
mean arterial blood pressure (MAP) 100

natural colloids 124, 128
albumin supplementation (*see* albumin)
clotting factors 27
plasma products 27
plasma products, types 26
protein particles 26
neuroendocrine mechanisms 107
neuroglycopenia 69
"Normal" saline 12
Normosol R and Plasma-Lyte 13
N-terminal probrain natriuretic peptide (NT-proBNP) 135

ocular disease 55
oncotic pressure 26; *see also* colloid osmotic pressure
osmotic demyelination syndrome (ODS) 119
osmotic nephrosis (ON) 22

packed cell volume and total protein (PCV/TP) 44, *99*
packed red blood cell transfusion (pRBC) 30
parathyroid hormone (PTH) 81
pediatrics/neonatals
adequate nutrition 130
age-related predisposing, critical illness **127**
assessment of sick 127
clinical case 131
compensatory mechanisms 126
extracellular fluid 126
fluid dosages 129–130
fluid loss 130
fluid types 127–128
hypoglycemia/hypokalemia 130–131
hypovolemia 126
jugular catheter, neck wrap *130*
maintenance fluid therapy 132
medical care 126
patients, metabolic demand 126
pediatric kitten for intraosseous access *129*
renal blood flow 127
resuscitation or rehydration 130

route of administration 128–129
subcategories 126
testing skin tent, ventral abdomen *128*
perioperative fluid therapy 115
peripheral catheters 34, *34*
point-of-care (POC) NT-proBNP ELISA tests 135
point-of care ultrasound (POCUS) 44, *50*, *99*
post-obstructive diuresis (POD) 138
potassium supplementation
balance 73
depolarization 73
clinical cases
ECF 73
hyperkalemia (*see* hyperkalemia)
intracellular 73
normal serum concentrations 73–74
protein-losing enteropathy 123
protein-losing nephropathy 123
pseudohyperkalemia 74
PTH *see* parathyroid hormone

red blood cell transfusion 46
renal blood flow (RBF) 110
renal disease *see* Acute kidney injury (AKI) and chronic kidney disease (CKD)
renal function 126
renal replacement therapy (RRT) 22
renin–angiotensin–aldosterone system (RAAS) 43, 56, 126
resting membrane potential (RMP) 73
restrictive (revised) approach 48–49, 98
"resuscitation rollercoaster" 98
routes of delivery
factors **34**
fluid therapy, phases 33
IV route 33
medical factors 33

semi-synthetic colloids
coagulopathy 21, 22
kidney injury *22*, 22–23
systemic inflammatory disease 23

sepsis
albumin volume 103
"appropriate" intravascular fluid replacement 104
balanced electrolyte solution 103
clinical cases 104–106
CPP 103, 104
definition 103
pathophysiology 103
septic shock 103, 104
sepsis/capillary leak syndromes 23
shock index (HR/SBP) 44
sodium bicarbonate 76
sodium–potassium adenosine triphosphatase (ATPase) pump 73, *74*, 77
subcutaneous administration (SC) 33
benefits/limitations **40**
canine patient, receiving SC fluids *39*
dehydration 38
disadvantages 39
fluid administration 38
gradual absorption 38
maintaining hydration 40
sympathetic nervous system (SNS) 43, *95*
syndrome of inappropriate ADH secretion (SIADH) 119
synthetic colloids 123, 128
albumin 18
COP 18
dextrans 18
gelatins 19
HES (*see* Hydroxyethyl starch (HES))
properties **19**
VetStarch *19*
synthetic/natural colloids 46

three-syringe technique 79
trauma-induced capillary leak syndrome 95
traumatic brain injury (TBI) 97, 101

urinalysis 57

vasopressin/anti-diuretic hormone 43
von Willebrand factor (vWf) 26